When Sex Isn't Good

[illegible]

[illegible]

[illegible]

When Sex Isn't Good

Stories & Solutions of Women With Sexual Dysfunction

Lillian Arleque, Ed.D.

Sue W. Goldstein, A.B.

Medical Consultant Irwin Goldstein, M.D.

iUniverse, Inc.
New York Lincoln Shanghai

When Sex Isn't Good
Stories & Solutions of Women With Sexual Dysfunction

iUniverse books may be ordered through booksellers or by contacting:

iUniverse
2021 Pine Lake Road, Suite 100
Lincoln, NE 68512
www.iuniverse.com
1-800-Authors (1-800-288-4677)

The information, ideas, and suggestions in this book are not intended as a substitute for professional medical advice. Before following any suggestions contained in this book, you should consult your personal physician. Neither the authors nor the publisher shall be liable or responsible for any loss or damage allegedly arising as a consequence of your use or application of any information or suggestions in this book.

ISBN: 978-0-595-42646-1 (pbk)
ISBN: 978-0-595-86973-2 (ebk)

Printed in the United States of America

For the husbands we love,
who provide us with passion and compassion,
sustenance and support.

Contents

Foreword by Irwin Goldstein, M.D. xiii

Preface xvii

Acknowledgments xix

Part I: The Stories

Frances' Story 3

Frances is a peri-menopausal woman who was distressed by her diminishing sexual function. She is an articulate woman who has chosen to share her story in many settings including public seminars and medical school classes.

Samantha's Story 9

Samantha is a thirty-six-year-old woman who has been married twice. She believed her first marriage failed because of her lack of sexual desire and the escalating sexual pain that she had hoped would be resolved through hysterectomy.

Diane's Story 19

Diane was diagnosed with diabetes in her late forties. As a later-in-life newlywed, she became distressed over her diminished sexual response, but her endocrinologist implied that it was "all in her head."

Lisa's Story 25

Lisa's childhood experience of sexual abuse resulted in her fear of close physical and emotional relationships. The anti-depressants prescribed throughout most of her adult life to help her cope with these issues exacerbated them as well, until she found help in her forties.

Olivia's Journal 31

Olivia had a plan. She had an out. She was not going to spend the rest of her life this way. At fifty, she had been diagnosed with persistent sexual arousal syndrome, and there was no cure.

Marie's Story 43

Marie, like Olivia, suffered from persistent sexual arousal syndrome, now called persistent genital arousal disorder. Communicating with other PSAS sufferers on the Internet became Marie's lifeline and a way to find resources to deal with her personal distress.

Leanne's Story 49

Leanne was happily married to a younger man and ready for sex as often as he was, until she reached forty-six. Her healthcare choices regarding her fibroid treatment were based on her desire to maintain a healthy sex life.

Debra's Story 55

Debra is a woman in her thirties with young children and pain so severe she was unable to look after them. Married to a man of few words, their communication dwindled because their relationship was more physical than verbal.

Irene and Harold's Story 61

Sexual dysfunction is a couple's issue. This is the story of a husband and wife in a long-term relationship in which each of the partners had to deal with sexual problems.

Elaine's Interview 67

Elaine is a thirty-nine-year-old woman whose sexual function was impacted by prolonged and debilitating pain. Her interview was so compelling that we chose to share some quotations taken directly from it.

Thea's Thoughts 73

Thea's relationship with her husband was deteriorating due to her lack of libido. She assumed her loss of interest in sex was the result of early menopause, but sought help because of the detrimental impact it was having on her marriage.

Trisha's Letter 79

Trisha is a peri-menopausal woman concerned about the future of her relationship because of her sexual health issues. Confused and vulnerable, she wanted to get better for her lover, as well as for herself.

Tracey's Story.......... 83

After being diagnosed as BRCA positive while still in her thirties, Tracey was forced to examine what lay ahead. Fortunately, she and her husband were able to make the difficult decisions together.

Lil's Story.......... 91

Lil, co-author of this book, lost her sexual desire at the age of twenty-nine, after giving birth to her first child. For over a quarter of a century, she went from doctor to doctor seeking a solution. In her fifties, Lil finally found a sexual medicine physician and confirmed what she knew all along, it wasn't "in her head," it was a biologic problem.

Sue's Story.......... 101

Sue is a fifty-five-year-old post-menopausal woman who is co-author of this book. Her story is about her transition through menopause. Each of her sexual health issues were resolved almost immediately because her husband is a sexual medicine physician.

Comments on Courtney.......... 109

In this story, the authors provide commentary on Courtney's situation. Her lack of knowledge of her sexual function was more common than most people would have believed, despite the plethora of available information about sex.

Part II: The Science

Sexual Medicine Overview by Irwin Goldstein, M.D.......... 115

Symptoms and Risk Factors by Irwin Goldstein, M.D.......... 121

Effects Of Medical Factors on Sexual Function by Irwin Goldstein, M.D..... 123

Anti-Depressants.......... 125

Cancer Treatment.......... 131

Childbirth.......... 139

Diabetes.......... 143

Hysterectomy.......... 147

Male Partner's Sexual Health.......... 153

Menopause.......... 163

Foreword

Dr. Irwin Goldstein is Director of Sexual Medicine, Alvarado Hospital, San Diego, California and Editor-in-Chief of The Journal of Sexual Medicine. Having practiced in the field of sexual medicine for over twenty-five years, he has authored more than three hundred twenty-five publications including books and chapters on different aspects of sexual dysfunction.

When Sex Isn't Good brings together stories of women of varied backgrounds and ages who have one thing in common—they have all been affected by sexual dysfunction and sought help from healthcare professionals. Their stories are both compelling and educational. The authors, well-respected individuals in their own fields, write from personal experience and have included their own unique stories.

In *When Sex Isn't Good*, true stories of women with sexual health concerns are told in a way that is gripping, powerful, and easy to understand. The identities of all the women whose stories are included in Part I have been changed for their privacy, except for the authors. In addition to an explanation of medical and psychologic factors affecting sexual function and therapies for sexual dysfunction in Part II, the Reference Section contains a glossary of terms and anatomical illustrations of a woman's genitalia. This material is meant not only to help you understand the stories, but to provide you with knowledge, language, and confidence to communicate effectively with your physician if you feel you have a sexual health concern that causes you distress. *When Sex Isn't Good* will empower you, and let you know that you are not alone.

Four out of ten women in the United States have sexual health problems, and approximately 25% of them have associated personal distress. Individuals with sexual health problems (and their partners) often lack education and knowledge about sexual medicine issues. One obvious consequence of this dearth of information is poor communication between members of the couple that can result in limited positive interaction between them. *When Sex Isn't Good* can provide a starting point for educational exploration of any sexual health concerns that may exist, or simply be an interesting collection of stories providing knowledge for future use.

Women are entitled to the same health standards as men—it should be "acceptable" for them to have a sexual health problem and to seek treatment without embarrassment or ridicule. A recent international consensus meeting reviewed rational and ethical evaluation and management strategies for women with sexual health concerns. You will read about some of these therapies and the choices made by the women whose stories are told in *When Sex Isn't Good.* It is important to note that while the first pharmacologic therapy has recently been approved in Europe by the EMEA, at this time there *does not exist* any FDA-approved pharmacologic treatment for women with sexual health problems.

Women are biologic and psychologic beings who do not live in a vacuum. Improved psychologic and biologic treatments for many sexual health problems are now being realized, geared toward the biologic, psychologic, and relational together or in parallel. The real question is, how does a woman receive this new sexual health care? A 760-page textbook on women's sexual health, *Women's Sexual Function and Dysfunction*, has recently been published. The vast majority of authors are members of the International Society for the Study of Women's Sexual Health (ISSWSH). The field of women's sexual health continues to develop, and members of ISSWSH are committed to its advancement.

Your gynecologist, primary care physician, or psychologist is the first line of intervention. She or he may be able to initially manage your sexual health problems. If appropriate, the second line of intervention is the sexual medicine physician. As presented in *When Sex Isn't Good*, the sexual medicine physician can explain why it may be preferable to change your anti-depressant as happened to Lisa, or the long-term effect on your sexual health of your having taken oral contraceptives when you were younger, as Thea experienced. The sexual medicine physician can help treat genital pain, as described by Elaine and Lil. Sue passed through menopause easily because her sexual medicine physician was able to promptly treat her symptoms, while Frances is hoping for the same outcome due to current management of her sexual health issues, and young women like Courtney may eventually be helped with a simple therapy.

The sexual medicine healthcare professional can help women like Diane, who is diabetic and became concerned about her diminished sexual response, and others like Olivia and her new friend Marie who had unrelenting, uncomfortable genital arousal. For some women like Irene, their problems seem to occur after their partners are treated. Sexual medicine specialists can work with the couple together. They are also able to work with other specialists, as is the case with Tracey where all treatments are chosen in conjunction with her oncologist.

When Sex Isn't Good informs and reminds the reader that women have the right to comprehensive health care, including sexual health care. This may include an appropriate level of sexual interest, satisfaction with sexual arousal, fulfillment with sexual orgasm, and sexual activity without accompanying sexual pain. If personal distress from your sexual health problem is causing you unhappiness, guilt, frustration, stress, feelings of inferiority, worry, inadequacy, regret, embarrassment, dissatisfaction or anger, you may wish to exercise your sexual health rights and seek treatment.

Women come in different shapes and sizes, as do their sexual health symptoms and solutions. *When Sex Isn't Good* is just a glimpse into some of the issues experienced by women of all ages, ethnicities, and socio-economic backgrounds. Share this book and share these stories with others. The educated woman is the empowered woman.

Irwin Goldstein, M.D.
Medical Consultant, *When Sex Isn't Good*

Preface

We the authors, both as women and as patients currently being treated for sexual dysfunction, wrote *When Sex Isn't Good* because we are passionate about the need for education in sexual medicine. Since people learn from the lives of others, we have chosen to compile a collection of interesting stories about real women who have struggled with symptoms of sexual dysfunction, and who have each made the decision to seek a solution for her sexual health concerns.

This book is a literary documentary, a collection of narratives developed through interviews with women who courageously volunteered to share their personal stories. They all did this so that you, the reader, would learn from their experiences and not endure the frustration and emotional distress of undiagnosed or untreated sexual dysfunction. In addition, we have incorporated an extensive science section into this book so that you might have a deeper understanding of the medical factors affecting sexual health as well as the therapies currently available.

When Sex Isn't Good is designed to inspire discussions between women and their partners, between women and their healthcare providers, and among women themselves. The other purpose of these stories is to educate women about their bodies and their sexual health. For that reason, we have chosen to include in Part II a sexual medicine overview, a list of symptoms and risk factors for sexual dysfunction in women, evidence-based scientific background information, and an explanation of various therapies. This section has been simplified for your use, however it includes references so that you may feel confidant sharing this with your physician.

The Reference Section contains a detailed glossary of terms to help you understand the science sections and easy-to-understand anatomical illustrations, all to empower you with the language necessary to discuss your sexual health concerns with your healthcare provider. We have even included a healthcare provider resource page.

Dr. Irwin Goldstein, noted sexual medicine physician, Director of Sexual Medicine, Alvarado Hospital, San Diego, California and Editor-in-Chief of *The Journal of Sexual Medicine*, served as medical consultant for this book.

Dr. Goldstein was responsible for the majority of the science included in Part II and the Reference Section, and for verification of the medical aspects of all stories in Part I.

Our personal stories represent the best and the worst of women's sexual health challenges. While Sue's sexual health issues were treated almost immediately, Lil sought care for twenty-seven years before she found a physician able to offer her a solution. It is our intent that after you read this book you will have the knowledge to articulate your symptoms and resources to seek your solutions for your sexual health concerns.

We have written this book for women and their partners because you need to know that you are not alone. Let it take you to a place you may not have been before, using language you may not have heard before, telling stories that may be your story, your sister's story, your mother's story or your daughter's. Furthermore, it is our wish that by helping to educate women, sexual health care will become available to all women everywhere.

Lil's Acknowledgments

To my husband Wayne: Throughout our almost forty years of marriage, you have continuously demonstrated the real meaning of unconditional love to our children and me. With courage and determination, you have faced a life filled with challenging health issues and yet, have selflessly put your own wants and needs aside for us. You constantly nurture my spirit and care for my physical needs, enabling me to focus my energies on my work and long term projects like this book. In spite of all my sexual health issues, your love and devotion for me never faltered. I am grateful and so deeply appreciative for you and your love—I know that I could have never achieved all that I have in my life if it wasn't for your never-ending support and encouragement, and I love you with all of my heart.

To my co-author Sue: The first time we met, I felt an immediate "soul" connection with you, and I knew that I *had* to get to know you. In my heart, I believe that this "connection" happened because we were meant to create something "bigger than ourselves." I call it destiny, you say it was "beshert" (thanks for all the Yiddish lessons.) We each brought our skills, knowledge, and backgrounds to this project, and in many wonderful ways, we were both compatible and complementary. Our work sessions not only helped us put this book together but also gave us the opportunity to share our lives and to build an incredible, lifetime friendship. It has been so much fun to work with you. I am really going to miss our "work" sessions and miss the time with you.… I guess this means we will have to write another book together!

To our medical consultant Dr. Irwin Goldstein: I never imagined when I first walked into your office that we would ultimately collaborate on a project that would change the lives of millions of women. Not only have you helped me regain my own sexual health, you have become a person whose friendship means the world to me. Over the last four years together, we have all laughed, vacationed, and solved many professional and personal problems. I have the utmost respect and admiration for who you are, and all that you do. It is an honor to know you and a blessing to be able to call you my friend.

To Kathleen and Jeff: You are, and continue to be, great gifts in my life. I have learned so much from you both. Kathleen, you are wise beyond your years, and I value your opinion and admire you for the kind of person you have become. You are the most incredible Mom to Elijah, and I watch you in awe when you interact with him. Jeff, I am so proud of your commitment to your country and community. You have been a teacher in my life. You have challenged me to become more than I ever thought possible. You have made me look at my own thoughts about myself and encouraged me to take risks. I know that you are both proud to call me your Mom and I am equally proud to say that you are my children. I love and adore you both with my whole heart.

To Elijah: Seeing your beautiful face, sweet smile, and unbelievable red hair reminds me of what is really important in my life.

To my mother Irene Duchesne: Thank you for all your love and encouragement and being there throughout my life—you are the BEST!

To my sister Katherine DeCesare: Thank you for moving in with Mom so she can live her last days at home. Doing this for her has allowed me to complete this book with focus and peace of mind.

To my niece Wendy: Thank you for your support and your many kindnesses to Grammy.

To Johanne: You have always been a great friend to me as I have attempted to "navigate" through my personal and professional challenges. I cannot express to you how much I value your many words of wisdom. Thank you also for your suggestions throughout the writing of this book—they were often "small" suggestions but they made a "big" difference.

To all my friends: Who knew that a girl who went to twelve years of Catholic schools would ever be writing a book about sex!! Thank you all for being in my life and for your support of this book.

To all my coaching clients: I have loved working with every one of you and I sincerely appreciate your interest in this book.

To Pat: You were such a positive influence in my life, teaching me to believe in myself, and encouraging me to go after my dreams. I will never forget you....

Sue's Acknowledgments

I want to thank family and friends
For their love and constant encouragement.
This project was hard work but we're at the end—
I just don't know where the time went!

First and foremost I have to thank
My steadfast friend and co-author, Lil,
Without whom this project would not have happened.
She gave support, guidance, and will.
She knew we could write a book to help
The many women who needed to learn
About their bodies and sexual function,
So she pushed me at every turn.

I also thank my daughter Lauren
Who helped us be more concise.
She hounded us to think of the reader
And wasn't always so very nice.
Her comments did allow us to grow
Through criticism, harsh but true,
Resulting in stories more interesting …
Better stories, just for you.

Thanks as well for support from the rest,
Andrew and Bryan (and Jaime his wife):
My children who are all out of the nest
And believed I could do this with my life.

Colleagues from ISSWSH have taught me much
But are far too numerous to mention here,
So I'll limit formal appreciation and such
To experts whose roles were very clear.

I want to extend my heartfelt thanks
To Sandra Leiblum whose expertise
In the field is well known, and who gave her time
To write about sex therapy, if you please.
Physical therapy references were written
By Talli Rosenbaum from Israel,
While that part was corrected in the stories by
Holly Herman, an expert as well.

If you turn to the back you'll see the work
Of Lori Messenger who supplied the art.
I am grateful that she took the time
To illustrate a woman's parts.
Another dear friend helped to critique
So I have to thank Linda Rosen
For taking the time to read and make comments
Although she didn't know why she was chosen.

The cover is by Jeremy Mack
Who took our thoughts and what we saw
And made great designs on front and back,
So thank you to my new son-in-law.

Irwin Goldstein wrote medical pages
Which are references in a never-ending part,
Providing information for all the ages;
Thank you and thank you from the bottom of my heart.

Deep thanks must be given, as well,
To the women willing to bare their souls
And tell their stories of symptoms and strife
So we could share their tales as a whole
Since, ultimately, the idea was a resource,
A book for you to find on the shelf
Of your local bookstore or on line

So each woman can help herself
With sexual healthcare that all deserve
But few have the language to talk with their doc.
I thank all of those who spoke with us
So that others might learn a lot.

From a personal place there are a few more
People whom I hold near and dear.
Although they may not have helped with the book, they
Helped me and therefore get mentioned here.
They are the oldest and youngest members
Of my family and I am glad
To throw kisses to my new grandson, Tyler,
And thank profusely my Mom and late Dad.

The last person on my list to cite
Is my husband of more than thirty years,
The man without whom I could not write,
And whom above all else I hold dear.
He taught me about sexual medicine, to
Believe in myself, and this book I could do.
So thank you, Irwin, I love you!

Part I

The Stories

Frances' Story

We had gone from being a young couple making love three times a week, to a middle-aged couple that hadn't touched each other in months.

Frances' Story

Frances is a peri-menopausal woman who was distressed by her diminishing sexual function. She is an articulate woman who has chosen to share her story in many settings including public seminars and medical school classes.

"Can we move your parents' beds together?" The nurses at the nursing home were concerned that my seventy-eight-year-old father would fall out of my mother's bed, so they were asking my permission to put their beds together. It seems my father was paying conjugal visits to my seventy-four-year-old mother on a regular basis. Knowing this, it was impossible for me to accept my physician's pronouncement that, at forty-three, *my* sex life was over.

When we married, Brian and I had a very active sex life, and neither one of us was embarrassed to enjoy it. Our sex life was fun—we had time to be crazy, time to pretend, time to play dress up and do stupid things. However, in my early forties sex just wasn't the same. I had lost my desire so I asked my doctor for help. He said this was an inevitable part of aging, but I could see a sex therapist if I wanted. I didn't bother because I didn't think that therapy would make a difference.

By my mid-forties I was in peri-menopause, and my focus was on housework and child rearing. Brian and I were beginning to feel more like brother and sister than husband and wife. As a couple, we had lost our playfulness. We both realized that something was different. My heart no longer raced when Brian came through the door. I was never shy, but I had become withdrawn. We didn't argue about sex, there was just a blandness in our relationship that made everything seem flat. I started dressing matronly—no reason to make myself attractive anymore. I became "beige." Sex became less and less frequent; it didn't interest me. It hadn't caused a problem in the relationship yet, but I imagined if it continued it could have led to divorce. You can't expect someone who is fully functional to be celibate.

Although I wasn't yet miserable, the night sweats and hot flashes drove me back to the doctor. To alleviate the symptoms, my primary care physician put me on birth control pills because my estrogen levels were low. He said that once the symptoms were gone, I might feel like having sex again. When I started to take the birth control pill, my night sweats and hot flashes did disappear. Unfortunately, my sexual response seemed to get worse, not better as my doctor anticipated. Brian and I rarely had sex, and when we did, it took longer for me to become aroused and to achieve orgasm.

After being on the pill for sixteen months, I had absolutely no desire, no arousal, no orgasm—nothing. We had gone from being a young couple making love three times a week, to a middle-aged couple that hadn't touched each other in months. Since you don't ask your friends how often they are having sex, we had no way of knowing whether the doctor was right when he said that this was part of aging. We were both frustrated and depressed.

When there is a problem in your life, you become receptive to any possible solutions, so when Brian and I saw a news report on television about a woman being treated for sexual dysfunction, I wrote down the name of her doctor. We decided right away to call for an appointment. We had already been through a lot of trying and crying; now we had hope again.

I was nervous going to see the sexual medicine specialist we had seen interviewed on television. My fear was that there would be no solution. You don't know if you're chasing after something that is impossible. I *was* getting older. I didn't expect Brian to stay with me simply because he felt he had to. I decided that no matter what the doctor said, I loved my husband enough to have sex with him more often even though the big thrill for me was gone.

The office visit was reassuring for both of us. The doctor was affable, very approachable, very upbeat, but clinical as well. He put us at ease. In addition to meeting with him and the staff psychologist, I had blood tests and a genital sensation test as part of my exam. My vaginal sensation was normal, but I had to wait for the results of the blood tests for my definitive diagnosis. On the way home, both of us were optimistic and excited. We have a car with a bench seat, and I sat in the middle next to Brian, something I hadn't done for years. We stopped at the drug store to pick up the lubricant the doctor had recommended, and I think we even had sex that night. It was reassuring to us that a physician believed that he could help us, and that we didn't have to accept my sexual dysfunction as a consequence of aging.

I felt good at my second appointment when I got the diagnosis. My blood tests indicated there really *was* something wrong, and it *could* be fixed. The first thing the doctor told me was that I should consider discontinuing oral contraceptives, because they were making my sexual problems worse. He started me on androgen therapy for the hypogonadism and local estrogen therapy for vaginal dryness and genital atrophy. Because he took the time to explain how the medications actually work, I was determined to adhere to my doctor's instructions for their use and for follow up blood tests.

It didn't take long for me to realize that the medications were making a difference. My clitoris felt more pliable and seemed a little more prominent. I don't think there was an exact moment when I realized it, but sex was getting better. It wasn't like when we were younger, but things definitely were better. I continued to feel changes in my body over the next couple of months. One day, I was sitting at my desk and felt tingling. I called Brian to tell him to come home right after work—for the first time in several years I felt desire. It's ironic that using male hormones made me feel more feminine.

My husband also noticed the change. I had more energy to do things with him, and no longer fell asleep on the couch in front of the TV. He was keenly aware that I was after him sexually. It felt like a reversal of roles when he said, "I have an early flight, so I have to get some sleep tonight."

Although my arousal and orgasm weren't what they used to be, they didn't have to be, because my ability to experience desire had returned to normal. When you feel good about yourself sexually, you feel good about all aspects of your life. It felt great to turn up the music in my car and drive my stick shift again. It felt wonderful to have desire again, but I worried whether this medication would keep working, so when I experienced peaks and valleys in my desire, I was afraid that it was going to disappear altogether, and I would be "beige" again.

The good news is there have been almost no side effects for me. I was concerned about hair loss because I have really fine hair. I do shed a little more now, but I have gone through periods in my life before when this has happened. I was worried about growing facial hair, but that hasn't been an issue. I was concerned about my skin, but my acne didn't get any worse. In retrospect, for me the side effects pale in comparison to the benefits from the treatment.

Despite the challenges with intimacy we faced in our marriage, my husband and I are once again enjoying our sex lives. *So there* to menopause! You didn't stop my mother, and you're not going to stop me. Brian and I plan to enjoy sex, even when *we* are in a nursing home.

To learn more about how menopause and oral contraception can affect sexual health and the therapies prescribed for Frances, refer to Part II: The Science.

Samantha's Story

I wouldn't even let him hold my hand because I didn't want him to interpret that as a sign that we could have sex.

Samantha's Story

Samantha is a thirty-six-year-old woman who has been married twice. She believed her first marriage failed because of her lack of sexual desire and the escalating sexual pain that she had hoped would be resolved through hysterectomy.

The drive into the city was uneventful. With no traffic problems to distract me, my thoughts about this appointment and what led me to it began to seep into my stream of consciousness. As I started to think about my life, and the many doctors' visits I'd been to, I realized that I was experiencing a weird combination of emotions—fear and trepidation as well as optimism and hope. After all, today could be the day that I would learn that my sexual relationship with my husband could be rejuvenated, or the day that, once again, another doctor would say that dreaded phrase, "Everything appears normal."

I became sexually active when I was almost sixteen. I had a lot of sex with numerous partners in college. I settled down in my junior year after meeting my future husband. We had a healthy sex life. Just after graduation, however, I was shocked to find out that I was pregnant. After having been on birth control pills for many years, I had switched to a cervical cap; that obviously hadn't worked. The thought of being a parent was truly terrifying because I was not emotionally ready. When I talked with my mother, her immediate response was to get an abortion. I agreed.

Six weeks into the pregnancy, three days before I was scheduled to start my first corporate job, I had an abortion. As emotionally difficult as it was, it was also physically problematic for me. At the time of my six-week follow-up visit I was still bleeding. My hormone levels were elevated, and it actually took three more months for the bleeding to stop. Once it did, I began to experience excruciating burning pain during intercourse. A laparoscopic examination determined I did not have endometriosis. My gynecologist said that the only explanation was that I "… must have been sexually abused as a child," and that my repression of it was the reason for the pain. That's when I decided to start therapy.

I have a close relationship with my mother, so I felt comfortable telling her about my pain during intercourse, and what the doctor had said. We both believed that since he was the doctor, he must know about these things. Her first response was to take out the photo albums with pictures of me as a child, so we could look for "some sort of something" that must have happened. After perusing the albums and much conversation in the family, my mother actually came up with the person that she believed might have molested me. In fact, because of what my gynecologist had said, my mother approached this relative and questioned him about possible abuse. Needless to say, all of this was extremely disruptive and destructive to my family.

Although therapy helped me with relaxation techniques for the stress, I stopped seeing the therapist because the counseling didn't reveal any evidence of sexual abuse. Yet, my fiancé and I continued to have problems with our sexual relationship. My pain with intercourse and resulting lack of desire inhibited intimacy and our ability to have a healthy sex life. We started to have doubts about whether or not we should get married. Trying to be positive about our future, and thinking that things would get better, we decided to go through with the wedding. Unfortunately, our hopes that our sexual problems would be resolved were never realized. We were married for two and a half years before we split up, and I don't think that we had intercourse more than fifteen times.

A few years later, I was fortunate enough to meet Rich. Since sex was good for the first two weeks of our relationship, I concluded that my past problems must have been a result of my not being in love with my ex-husband. It wasn't long, however, before things went downhill. My problems with lack of desire and pain had not gone away—they seemed to get worse. I remember many days when I would cry out of frustration and pain. Now, I wasn't just having pain with intercourse; the discomfort would persist for two days afterward. In addition, I began to feel like I had a chronic yeast infection because there was always a dull burning in my vaginal area. The only way I was able to function was by wearing loose clothing. I even stopped wearing underwear because it seemed to make the burning worse. I went to the doctor frequently, believing I had a recurrent yeast infection, but the lab results always came back normal. The pain became so intense that I actually examined myself with a mirror. What I saw scared me to death—sores in my vaginal area! The doctor diagnosed it as herpes. I was so upset … how could that have happened? When the blood work came back negative for herpes, the doctor reexamined me only to find the sores were gone. He had no explanation, but said that everything appeared normal and to come back if the sores returned. So what was wrong with me, and what were the sores?

All of these problems had a detrimental impact on our relationship. Rich and I had many discussions about it, yet he stayed with me, even when my problems became more complicated. In 1996, I started bleeding heavily. Since there was a history of fibroid tumors in my family, I requested an ultrasound. The doctor felt this unnecessary because he hadn't detected any fibroids during his examination. Instead, he put me back on birth control pills. Not only was I having problems with lack of desire and pain with intercourse, I was now having difficulty with lubrication that I assumed related to being on the pill.

I was still having vaginal bleeding three years later, so I changed doctors. I had blood work done the week before my physical exam with the new doctor. At 10:30 that night, when I was home alone, the phone rang. It was the doctor from the blood lab calling me to find out if I had had my blood drawn because of chest pains, which was a surprise since I was feeling fine. He proceeded to tell me that my hemoglobin count was six, and that I could go into cardiac arrest at any time, so I better call my doctor first thing in the morning. I was terrified. When I saw my doctor the next day, she said that the report must have been a mistake—this couldn't be my blood work. I had so much color from my recent trip to Aruba, the doctor was shocked when she turned my tanned hands over and discovered my palms were colorless. I had been bleeding all this time, and no one had paid any attention to the consequences. I finally had an ultrasound and was diagnosed with a fibroid tumor. Being reluctant to have surgery, I opted to try iron shots first. Three blood transfusions later, I finally agreed to undergo a hystoscopic myomectomy. My recovery went well, but by the end of the year I was bleeding heavily again. I had no interest in sex, but justified my lack of desire because I was disgusting—bloody and gross all the time. Two years after the first surgical procedure, I gave in and had a hysterectomy.

Rich and I had been together for six years before we married, but our sexual relationship had never been ideal. Sometimes he would get frustrated about our lack of sex, but then he would see what I was going through. Rich would support me and say, "I know we'll get through this." He was by my side through all of the procedures and asked me to marry him one month after my hysterectomy. He was probably thinking, now we could have sex because all the obvious physical problems appear to have been eliminated. When I recovered and still didn't have desire for sex, we talked about it. I felt that perhaps a lot of the earlier issues around desire were recurring, or that my lack of desire resulted from not being able to have sex for so long. Looking back, I realize that I hadn't desired sex for fifteen years. Now, there were no more excuses not to, so we had sex more often.

While the hysterectomy stopped the bleeding, the vaginal pain persisted. Rich could see it on my face and he would say, "I'm hurting you, I'm hurting you!" Whenever I questioned doctors about the pain, the response was that I needed to use more lubrication. We used a lot of lubrication when having intercourse to diminish the pain, but the day after, my vagina would feel like it was on fire. We couldn't have sex for the next few days because the thought of it was just unbearable.

Through all of this, I felt so alone. I had mentioned the pain to my mother when the issue of abuse came up, but I never talked to her about the kind of pain and the intensity. When I got together with my girlfriends, they would talk about the great sex they were having, and I would lie and say, "Yeah, me too." I remember one friend, in particular, talking about her sex life and how she said she had never said "No" to her husband. I was like, "*Never?*" In that kind of environment, where my friends were talking about how they did it every night and loved it, I wasn't going to say I didn't. These experiences affirmed for me that something was really, really wrong. I had reached out to physicians and psychologists, and nobody was able to help me. I was extremely discouraged and at a loss about what to do next.

It's funny how life works. Just when you think there's no solution in sight, you get a glimmer of hope. In talking with one of my closest friends about my sexual problems, she told me that her aunt went to a sexual medicine physician. My friend said, "You need to see him." At the time, I had numerous excuses for not making the appointment, but I realize now that it was because of my anxiety. I was scared that if I went, I was going to find out that I was "normal," and that the problem was "all in my head." As bizarre as it sounds, I thought if I didn't go, I could hold on to the fact that something was physically wrong. I had the phone number for more than a year, and still wouldn't have called if my friend's aunt hadn't asked me to help out with registration for a public seminar on Female Sexual Dysfunction, where the sexual medicine specialist was speaking. I didn't know at the time, but my friend and her aunt had collaborated to get me there.

A lot of my concerns were alleviated at the seminar. I listened to the lecture on sexual dysfunction in women, and to the patients telling their stories, and realized that there were women out there just like me. As I looked around the room at the more than two hundred attendees, my first thought was that probably half the population is suffering in some way from sexual dysfunction. The media bombards us daily with sexual images that make those of us with sexual dysfunction feel inadequate, and therefore less likely to talk about our sexual problems. I wondered how many people have sex, in spite of the pain, just to make someone else happy. I've done it. I've had sex with my husband despite my pain, just so he doesn't feel like he has to jump off a bridge. How many women have pain and no desire, yet their husbands expect them to have sex all the time? It is all so sad.

After the seminar was over, I talked with one of the women on the patient panel. She described how she avoided having sex, and I could identify with that. It was such a relief to know that I wasn't alone, that other women were going through the same thing, and there might be hope for me. There is so much love between my husband and me, but I did everything I could to avoid Rich touching me. I have always craved intimacy, being able to hug, snuggle, and kiss, but I totally cut myself off from that because I knew where it could lead. I put up this wall. I wouldn't even let him hold my hand because I didn't want him to interpret that as a sign that we could have sex.

Inspired by the seminar, I made an appointment with my primary care doctor. I had been there several weeks earlier and had gone through my medical history, but I never mentioned the issue of my sexual dysfunction. I wanted to have that discussion with her, even though this would be an emotional conversation for me, because the last time I mentioned my sexual problems to a physician, he recommended therapy for sexual abuse.

Having attended the seminar, I knew to go to the sexual medicine clinic's Web site and download the list of recommended blood tests. I asked my primary care doctor to write the prescription for the lab work and to send the actual lab report directly to me, so that I could have it for my appointment at the clinic. On December 24th, I received a letter from my doctor stating that the blood test results were normal, and therefore there was no need for me to seek further consultation. So I decided I would cancel my appointment. While on vacation the following week, I was in so much pain that I knew I had to keep the appointment, in spite of what my doctor said. When we returned from our trip, I requested the actual lab results. I tried to read them but they didn't make any sense to me. The letter said that I was normal, so once again I almost cancelled my appointment. When I mentioned that to my friend, she talked me out of it. I would go, but I was really scared.

Although my drive to the hospital was easy, as I got closer I got even more nervous. My fear was that this sexual medicine physician was going to tell me that I was "normal," that there was nothing really wrong with me. And I was afraid that, once again, I was going to feel stupid and humiliated.

When I couldn't find a parking space, I started to panic. I wished that my husband were with me, but he had been unable to come because of his work schedule. I finally parked and went inside. Filling out the paperwork in the office helped distract me from my fears and emotions. When I met with the psychologist in the clinic, I explained that I had been medicated for depression on and off since 1993 and finally found the right anti-depressant about five years ago. I learned at the seminar that some anti-depressants could cause sexual dysfunction.

When I finished talking with the psychologist, she brought me in to meet the doctor. He made me feel comfortable and safe talking about the intimate details of my sex life. I could sense his caring and eagerness to help. He had a great sense of humor that helped put me at ease, in contrast to my previous health-care professionals, but I was anxious about what he was going to say regarding the blood work. I just wanted to get it over with. I handed him the results and told him that my doctor said they were normal. He flipped the paper around to show the normal ranges for free testosterone. "Do you see what yours says? Do you know what that means? It means it's unreadable. Less than .5 is too small to read. Your results are *not* normal." He also showed me that my sex hormone binding globulin levels were elevated, and explained how that contributed to my sexual dysfunction. I felt so validated. For fifteen years, I had been trying to figure out what was wrong with me, when I had been told repeatedly that nothing was wrong, it was "in my head." Now that I knew I would need hormones, just let me go home and start taking them.

I had an answer, and I knew what was wrong with me, but we weren't done yet. The second part of the visit was a physical exam including sensation testing. I assumed the results would be normal—we had already figured out the problem. This test determines the level of perception to a vibration stimulus that is placed on your genitals, in comparison to your finger. The results indicated that I had minimal sensation. The ideal is three volts, and I required twelve volts before I could feel it. Now it made sense why I needed my husband to press so hard. He wanted to be gentle because of the pain I experienced, yet because of my low sensitivity, I needed him to get "rough" so I could feel something, which caused me days of pain afterward.

Finally, I knew my sexual dysfunction was a result of a lack of available testosterone and low vaginal sensitivity. When the doctor examined me, he discovered that the hood of my clitoris would not retract, my labia minora were partially fused to the labia majora, and numerous minor vestibular glands around the vaginal opening were inflamed. This was what the gynecologist must have seen when he thought I had herpes. The sexual medicine physician said that, based on the physical changes that he saw, it was clear that this problem had been going on for a long time. He explained to me how my lack of available testosterone could have diminished my vaginal sensation, making it hard to be aroused during intercourse. It could also have caused the inflammation and the intense pain I had been experiencing. He asked me about the pain scale I had completed earlier. When you have been living with pain for such a long time, you survive by not thinking of it. The pain wasn't excruciating at the time of my exam, but my vaginal area never felt quite right. I especially noticed it when I had been sitting for a long time, and I fidgeted to try to feel more comfortable. I was constantly aware of that part of my body, and that I didn't want to be touched there. The doctor then took a Q-tip and started touching the glands. I nearly hit the ceiling. With tears in my eyes I screamed, "Oh my God. That's the same burning feeling that I have for two days after I have sex."

I left the appointment feeling this incredible sense of relief, but soon these emotions turned into anger. I was angry with my previous physicians and disappointed with my new gynecologist. As a female physician who believed in holistic medicine, I thought that she was "the best of the best." Why hadn't she noticed the physical changes in my vaginal area? Why hadn't she told me that a hysterectomy could affect my sexual function? The sexual medicine specialist told me not to get angry but to educate her.

There is no doubt in my mind that my sexual dysfunction was probably the reason for the break up of my first marriage. It amazes me that my relationship with my second husband has survived all of this chaos. I have wished so many times that I would never have to have sex again. There were times when I was so distraught, I would tell Rich that it was okay to go elsewhere if he really needed it. I think the only reason that our relationship and our marriage have survived all of this was because we communicated openly about the issues.

I am grateful to have found a sexual medicine physician who listened to me, understood what was wrong, and offered a solution for my problems. Now, two years later, I continue to use the androgen therapy he prescribed and work with my primary care physician to make sure all my blood values stay normal. And Rich and I are still happily married.

To learn more about how anti-depressants, hysterectomy, oral contraception, and vulvodynia can affect sexual health and the therapies prescribed for Samantha, refer to Part II: The Science.

Diane's Story

The thought of discussing my sex life with a sexual medicine physician just terrified me.

Diane's Story

Diane was diagnosed with diabetes in her late forties. As a later-in-life newlywed, she became distressed over her diminished sexual response, but her endocrinologist implied that it was "all in her head."

My first husband had an affair with my best friend. I was traumatized, in total shock. I was *still* in therapy ten years later when I met Nick.

After a six-year courtship we married, and at forty-eight I never dreamed that I could be so happy. Life was wonderful, sex was great, and everything seemed perfect until six months after our wedding, when I was diagnosed with insulin-dependent diabetes.

Over time, I learned to manage my diabetes. What I couldn't handle was its eventual negative impact on my sex life. Where I had been multi-orgasmic in the past, I now only occasionally experienced orgasm from intercourse. The only way I could regularly climax was with oral sex. After fifteen years of marriage, I was willing to have intercourse with Nick to satisfy him, but I wasn't willing to pretend. Sex was no longer the pleasurable experience for me that it once was because I wasn't feeling any sensation. We had many discussions about this problem because sex was important to both of us. Being a kind and loving person who likes to fix things, my husband was frustrated because he couldn't figure out how to fix this or make sex better for me.

In researching diabetes and sexual dysfunction, I found countless information about diabetic men and impotence but virtually nothing written about sexual problems in diabetic women. The endocrinologist treating my diabetes implied my sexual problem was "in my head." Since I couldn't find any good information on the topic, I was convinced the doctor was correct. When I met with the nurse educator at the diabetes clinic, I decided to ask her about diabetic women and sexual function. She recommended I make an appointment with a specialist. The thought of discussing my sex life with a sexual medicine physician just terrified me. "I'm going to discuss *this* with a stranger? What *is* a sexual medicine doctor?" I put the doctor's number in my desk drawer hoping that I would never have to make the call, and Nick never pressured me to do it.

We tried our best to maintain some normalcy in our relationship. We went along, focusing on things we enjoyed doing together, but we both missed the sexual satisfaction that was an integral part of our relationship. I was still willing to satisfy Nick whenever he approached me despite my lack of interest, however, when I was giving him pleasure my mind was on other things ... what I was going to prepare for dinner ... what I was going to wear to work....

Eventually, I could not reach orgasm at all with sexual intercourse, bringing me to tears. Every now and then, I would climax with oral sex, so maybe the endocrinologist *was* right, and my problem *was* all in my head. Or, I would think that it was something that I wasn't doing, and Nick would think it was something he wasn't doing. Although I wasn't worried about Nick straying, in the back of my mind I had nagging doubts. It is a tribute to my husband that he never gave up on me because over that year things significantly worsened. Out of desperation, I pulled open my desk drawer and searched for the telephone number of the sexual medicine physician.

It was hard for me to go to the sexual medicine doctor because I thought my problem was psychologic. Just making the call had been a traumatic experience. The first time I went to see him I was really nervous. I've never had a healthcare provider ask me specifically about my sexual health. After all my interviews, my physical exam, and a review of my blood test results, he informed me that I had the hormonal blood values of a five-year-old. I burst into tears of relief—it was not in my head, it was in my body. And even now my eyes well up when I think about it. It was my body....

As we left the clinic, Nick said that he was proud of me because he didn't think that he could have been so open. What he didn't realize was the depth of my desperation. At that point, I would have done anything reasonable to regain my sexual function. The fact that I had a strong desire to restore my sexual health meant a lot to Nick, and this helped bring us closer together in spite of the problems we were having.

It took a long time—almost a year—but my sexual function was returning. I needed to be conscientious with my medications and blood tests, and gradually things started coming back. It had been almost two years since I had experienced a real orgasm. The first time I had an orgasm again, during oral sex, was such an emotional event that I cried. I continued taking all the medications prescribed by my sexual medicine doctor, and eventually began to have orgasms with intercourse. The first time *that* happened, we wanted to open a bottle of champagne and celebrate!

It is not clear in my mind whether or not menopause caused the sexual problems. For me, menopause was nothing. I am convinced that most of my problems were caused by diabetes. There is a lot of good literature about men with diabetes and erectile dysfunction, but almost nothing about women with diabetes and sexual health problems. My endocrinologist said biologic sexual dysfunction from diabetes is more of a male thing, but I realize from my own experience that's not really true; there just isn't a lot written on this topic yet.

I had been so nervous to talk about my sexual health in the past, but when I recently went to my gynecologist for my annual exam, she and her nurse were both open to hearing me talk about sexual dysfunction and learning more about it. I've talked to my friends about this, and the more I talk about it, the more comfortable I feel talking about it. I am hoping to help educate people about sexual health. I've come to realize that in spite of my diabetes, I can have an active sex life. I've made a commitment to myself to be as faithful with all of my sexual health medications as I am with my diabetes medication. I still haven't reached where I was sexually before this happened, the improvement has been gradual, but things are much better now. And I've come to the conclusion that I am not alone.

To learn more about how diabetes and menopause can affect sexual health and the therapies prescribed for Diane, refer to Part II: The Science.

Lisa's Story

I should have believed in myself, instead of letting everyone else tell me that my problems were "all in my head."

Lisa's Story

Lisa's childhood experience of sexual abuse resulted in her fear of close physical and emotional relationships. The anti-depressants prescribed throughout most of her adult life to help her cope with these issues exacerbated them as well, until she found help in her forties.

Despite my fears about having sex and attempts to avoid relationships with men, strangely, I am still attracted to them.

I know that, as a child, I was not what you would call "normal." I have vague memories of being sexually abused at six. *Not* by my dad, although there were times when his behavior made me feel uncomfortable. I think my fears and lack of security must have been manifested through nightmares. They eventually became so bad that my parents once took me to a child psychiatrist, although my mother has since denied the fact.

By the time I was twenty-one, I was depressed and feeling anxious much of the time. My doctor put me on a medication that would relieve my depression, but I felt so drugged I used it for less than a year. Throughout my twenties, I saw several therapists and was prescribed a variety of medications, including an anti-anxiety drug, an anti-depressant, and a drug to help me focus. I had always explored my body as a child, and as a young adult, I enjoyed stimulating my clitoris until I reached orgasm. I had absolutely no sexual desire in my twenties when I was on the anti-depressant. Yet, I needed those medications just to function. They didn't provide a great quality of life, but without the drugs I would burst into tears over nothing. I had panic attacks, heart palpitations, and a tremor in my voice, especially in social situations around men.

I was still a virgin in my mid-twenties when I had my first vaginal exam and Pap smear. The doctor couldn't even get his finger in, let alone a speculum! That was the first time I became aware of feeling sharp pain from insertion. I told the doctor I had stopped wearing tampons in my early twenties. It always felt like the tampon was half in, half out, and when I asked my friends about it, they said tampons didn't bother them. I just assumed it was me, and that I was odd. The gynecologist suggested that I stretch my vagina, but it was too painful to even consider. I went for a few gynecologic exams over the next fifteen years and had the same problem each time. One gynecologist told me I had vaginismus, and that the problem was psychological, so he recommended I see a therapist. No amount of therapy resolved the pain problem, and I was still a virgin.

At thirty-four, I changed careers and became a flight attendant. As I was traveling all the time, I was able to see different doctors and therapists in a variety of locations. My confidence was so low that I believed everything they said—they were smarter than me—that the problem *was* "in my head." They wouldn't treat me beyond prescribing anti-depressants. Even if my pain was psychological, no one dealt with the actual physical discomfort that I had with insertion. I finally went to a physician who specialized in vaginismus. When even she couldn't manage my pain, I sought alternative therapies. I tried trigger point injections of local anesthesia for the pain and switched to acupuncture for the depression and anxiety, but they didn't help. I needed to deal with my depression and treat the pain, but when I returned to the counselor, she wanted to put me back on a selective serotonin reuptake inhibitor. I knew from experience that an anti-depressant only served as a bandage for one problem and created another. I started looking into herbs, and I was seeing still another counselor. One caring doctor gave me the name of a physical therapist but since she didn't explain how the therapist could help me, I didn't go.

Around this time I read an article about a sexual medicine doctor near my home. My therapist didn't feel that the doctor could help, but I decided to start taking control of my life and made an appointment anyway. I remember wondering why this doctor would be any different …

… I sat down and the doctor talked with me, making it clear that I didn't need to be embarrassed. Treating my vagina was like treating any other part of the body. He put on these funny goggles to examine me and immediately saw the problem. His were the first hopeful words that I had heard in decades. He touched different areas around my labia with a cotton swab, and I was supposed to tell him how much pain I was in, on a scale from one to ten. Where the vaginal pain was a "seven," he gave me a shot of a local anesthetic, and the pain disappeared. When the medication wore off later, it felt like I had been kicked in the crotch. All those years I had been misdiagnosed because no one had looked under the speculum at my vestibule. Now I had a diagnosis of vulvar vestibulitis syndrome.

The nurse took some blood, and I came back a few weeks later to talk about the results. The doctor explained that I had the androgen levels of a pre-pubescent child. He started asking me many questions trying to figure out why my androgens were low, but all I can remember now is that I told him I had never taken birth control pills, although I had been on selective serotonin reuptake inhibitors for a significant number of years.

He started me on androgen therapy, and my depression lifted for the first time in five years; I hadn't been on anti-depressants for all that time. Then I had conservative surgery to remove the painful lesion in my vestibule. The pain had been an "eight" prior to surgery, but lowered to a "five" afterward. The doctor planned a second surgery to try to eliminate the remaining pain. This time he removed the bottom four glands. After the second surgery healed I was pain free. I went for a Pap smear and was thrilled to actually have my gynecologist complete the exam.

Now I am peri-menopausal. I go back to my sexual medicine doctor when he takes my blood to check my hormone levels. I am on dehydroepiandrosterone and testosterone gel and local estrogen, and that has really helped. He also started me on a dopamine agonist for my depression and libido.

I am furious with the psychology community for trying to convince me that the pain was "in my head" because of my childhood abuse. They should have supported me and encouraged me as I sought alternative solutions. I wish the first time I had gone into a doctor's office for my pain I had felt more confident in my knowledge of my own body. I should have believed in myself, instead of letting everyone else tell me that my problems were "all in my head." If I had believed in myself, my doctors may have believed me. I should have shared my story with my family as well, so that they could have supported me when I had my surgery. I didn't bring it up because I thought they would have been uncomfortable. Now I know better. Like the doctor said, it's just another part of the body.

Even though the reason for the physical pain was solved, I was still carrying a fear that I didn't know how to address. For more than twenty years I had been trying to isolate myself, protect myself. I had been mentally and emotionally shielding myself from men and the vaginal pain that might come with intimacy. But I wanted to develop a relationship with a man, get married, and have children some day. And now in my early forties, I am trying to learn how to be intimate in a relationship; I am just starting to figure out the difference between boundaries and barriers.

Now comes the real work. I can see a change in myself already, but I don't think anyone else can. Since my sexual issues have been resolved, I am feeling better, finally taking care of my needs, and optimistic about my future. I am no longer afraid of having a relationship with a man.

To learn more about how anti-depressants and vulvodynia can affect sexual health and the therapies prescribed for Lisa, refer to Part II: The Science.

Olivia's Journal

I think I might as well accept the fact that my good life is over—
I really should have ended my life three years ago.

Olivia's Journal

Olivia had a plan. She had an out. She was not going to spend the rest of her life this way. At fifty, she had been diagnosed with persistent sexual arousal syndrome, and there was no cure.

6/7/02
Prospect of life like this for another 40 years is a complete nightmare, and something I refuse to face. I have always taken good care of myself, so how did this happen to me? My sex drive is a tyrannical, unrelenting, hyped-up caricature of normal, 24/7/365. Hard to concentrate on anything else, difficult to grin and pretend to be okay. Sleep is nearly impossible. Life is horrible. Paul and I still have sex about 3 times a week when he's home, but I have to masturbate every single day to try to relieve some of the tension. Orgasms are strangely incomplete, and my need for sexual release sometimes returns immediately, sometimes a few hours later. I was absolutely fine and sex was great until I was 47.

8/2/02
I constantly feel aroused—the throbbing in my genitals never stops, and all I want to do is have an orgasm to feel better. Now, I even have trouble reaching orgasm, despite the perpetual need. I can't live this way.

8/11/02
It has been hard to muster up the courage to explain to my psychiatrist all of my symptoms because he is about 15 years younger than me and really good-looking. Our entire conversations have focused on my life-long depression. I think if I take Paul along with me, I won't be so embarrassed to talk about my sexual issues. I am pretty sure that the problem is related to the medication that I'm on. I haven't told my psychiatrist because I like the way the anti-depressant makes me feel, so I've just put up with having lousy sex for a long time.

8/12//02
Paul and I sat with my psychiatrist today and explained what has been happening. I described my symptoms to him, how I have been climbing the walls. It started about the time I could no longer reach orgasm. It seemed like pressure was building from that, and if I could just come I wouldn't feel aroused all the time. I was perfectly normal—what made my body change? At least now I think I know what I have. My psychiatrist just read an article on persistent sexual arousal syndrome, and thought that might be it. I think I *do* have PSAS because it is perpetual. Whatever it's called, I just need to get rid of it.

8/19/02
The psychiatrist stopped one medication, tried another, but that just made it worse. This has to end—I can't live like this. My doctor is floundering.

10/23/02
I traveled out of state for this big deal consultation. This was a sexual behavior clinic but I was so desperate that I didn't give a damn. Paul came with me because they do it as a couple. They had pretty much nothing to offer, except they suggested that it was a manic manifestation, and that I could try an anti-seizure medication and maybe ECT. That's the first time that I'd heard about that as a possibility. ECT's are pretty serious stuff. It's electroconvulsive therapy, where they put electrodes on your skull—I'll have to think about it.

11/19/02
I got a referral today for a far more experienced psychiatrist. I desperately need help. My day-to-day living is horrible. I can't do the things I love—gardening, gourmet cooking, walking my dog....

2/06/03
I went to see a neuropsychiatrist today who is an expert in ECT. I felt comfortable with him, and he seems to know what he is talking about.

2/13/03
Paul came with me today to Dr. K's office, to be there with me to hear my treatment options. I asked Dr. K about ECT, since the expert at the other clinic suggested this as a possible therapy. I was relieved when he said no, ECT's are pretty drastic. He seems to think that my constant arousal may have something to do with mini-seizures and wants to try anti-seizure medicine first.

2/14/03
Paul and I talked today about my options. I don't have a choice. I can't live like this, and I'm afraid of the shock treatments. I will ask Dr. K at my next visit to prescribe the anti-seizure medicine. But I'm a little nervous about that too....

4/10/03
I will not give up until I find an answer. Today, I went to a sex therapist a friend recommended. She couldn't help, but gave me the name of a urologist. I'll call him tomorrow.

4/11/03
I lucked out! He had a cancellation. I see him in 2 weeks. I have a really good feeling about this.

4/25/03
Bad news—good news. The urologist was really nice, but he didn't have a clue. He did, however, give me the name of a sexual medicine specialist. I got home too late today to call. I have to wait until Monday to make an appointment.

7/10/03
I finally saw Dr. G this morning. It seems like months since I got his name from that urologist. Now, I have a second diagnosis of female sexual dysfunction. FSD, PSAS, these acronyms are getting discouraging. He drew blood—I hope he has some answers for me on my next visit.

8/15/03
Dr. G showed me my lab results today. Now I have to use DHEA, testosterone gel, and an estrogen pill that I put in my vagina. It's been 10 years since I went through menopause. These new medications are supposed to make my hormones normal again so I can have orgasms and get some relief from the constant throbbing. He also got the okay from Dr. K to increase my anti-seizure medication.

9/1/03
I feel better on the anti-seizure medicine and am pretty happy right now. I hope that the new FSD meds will help me reach orgasm again. That's what Dr. G hopes too.

10/4/03
While the anti-seizure medication helps life remain tolerable, I think the FSD medications are finally working. Last night I had my first orgasm in ages. I know from other members of a PSAS online support group that having orgasms doesn't always help, but for me they are a real blessing.

11/30/03
Now that Dr. G has straightened out my hormones, I am starting to get "spontaneous orgasms." The constant level of sexual tension is so high, it spontaneously bubbles over into something that can only be described as a form of orgasm, no matter what I'm doing. But they are muted and ineffective as far as bringing relief. They are distracting and cause embarrassing blushing and facial twitching, just another part of a really hideous syndrome.

4/11/04
I barely survived Easter services. I need Dr. G! I can't wait for him to increase my anti-seizure medication once again, so I can make it through another day.

8/9/04
The anti-seizure medicine immobilizes me. All I can accomplish is what I prioritize first—work. The PSAS still has not resolved completely, but it's down to a dull roar; I can live with that, sort of. I gained 40 pounds already, but I don't care, because who wants to live with PSAS anyway. I would much rather treat my genitals, get off the horrible drug, and simply take an anti-depressant for the brain. To hell with sex!

8/19/04
I survive, and that's the only way to describe it, on more than 10 times my original dose of that damn medicine. It's been over a year now. I am miserable from the sluggishness and the residual PSAS symptoms. The weight gain, the puffiness, the facial grimacing, the depression are overwhelming me. Dr. K wants me to have ECT. I know he is supposed to be an expert, but what they know about it is very crude, and I am really concerned about memory loss. If it were not for the PSAS, I could go on a plain old anti-depressant and be done with it.

2/8/05
I'm afraid that I was too optimistic that I could have a future. I hate the side effects of the anti-seizure medicine so, so much. I've gained about 45 lbs, not from overeating but from hardly moving. The stuff makes me a zombie. I've

tried to get off it, but each time the PSAS roars back and is not one bit better than it was before. My psychiatrist had hoped that it would stop, but it didn't. Is there any hope at all? Dr. K wants to do ECT but I am afraid. All I can think of is the stuff that I saw in the old Frankenstein movie. I have suffered for more than 3 years. I am thinking about just ending it all. I need relief. Cremation *will do it.*

2/9/05
I thought I was getting better. My PSAS *never* goes away, it is not episodic, never relieved except with that goddamn medication. I think I might as well accept the fact that my good life is over—I really should have ended my life 3 years ago. I need this fixed *now*. This is hell on earth and I refuse to live like this. I may do the ECT because it seems that no one has tried that, but I have promised myself that if that doesn't completely relieve it, I will end this. I expect to be the first recorded PSAS suicide.

2/11/05
Yesterday, I had my pre-anesthesia workup and my neuropsychiatric testing for my upcoming ECT. This is an extreme treatment for an extreme problem. No one has ever tried it for PSAS, but I don't have a lot to lose. I am terribly depressed, but all of the anti-depressants make this worse. I have told Dr. K that this *will* end, one way or another. He understands. I have to get out of this living hell. I regret not having killed myself 3 years ago. So this looks like my only shot. I start Monday, Feb 14. Valentine's Day—ironic.

2/18/05
So far so good. It actually does seem to be helping after 3 treatments, but I'm afraid to get my hopes up.

2/23/05
My PSAS is just about gone, and I can't believe it. Paul says I have more memory loss than I am aware of, so I'm sticking close to home.

2/25/05
The treatments make me forget a few things, but my memory comes back each time after a few days. In any event, it is certainly worth it.

2/27/05
The PSAS symptoms are completely gone. Dr. K suggested I go with maintenance ECT's. It will be hard to get away from work for a whole day, so I'm

hoping I can just forget about them if I don't have a relapse. I never thought I would be normal again. It is like being reborn. I have rejoined the human race. Paul and I have been married 28 years, and he is quite glad to have me back. He is very grateful to my doctors. Whatever was wrong with my brain seems to have been reversed by ECT. I am so happy to be able to walk the dog—that used to be very hard with the PSAS. Now that I'm moving again, I've lost the first 10 pounds.

2/28/05
Paul is so happy that I am back to normal. I've done the ECT, and I continue to take the medicines Dr. G prescribed. We're making love on Paul's schedule—about 3 times a week. With my arousal and orgasm back to normal, a statement I *never* thought I would get to make again, I love making love.

3/4/05
I always wonder whether the hypogonadism preventing orgasm may have created a kind of back pressure making everything that much worse—certainly that's how it felt. If I had talked to my young psychiatrist earlier, would it have made a difference? I feel guilty about that. I feel like my crotch is gradually becoming more and more normal.

3/14/05
It's back … ECT tomorrow … I wonder how practical it is going to be to do what is called maintenance ECT, and whether they will be able to do enough to keep the "monster" at bay. I am *not* going to live like this. I have an exit strategy and will use it if needed. Life should have a basic quality to it.

3/16/05
I am quite a bit better today. This ECT and small dose of anti-seizure medication really works for me. The kinks have to be worked out, but at least there is something to work with. This is still the best quality time I have had in over 3 years.

3/31/05
I saw Dr. K in his office, and he didn't change anything. I stopped the anti-seizure medicine, last dose Tuesday night, and even though it is such a tiny amount, it does do something because I woke up (early) this am with the PSAS that has flourished as the day has gone on. Tomorrow am, ECT.

4/1/05
Today was pretty rough. The other times I had no real side effects, but this time I toughed it out with no medicine for 2 days before. Dr. K was pleased because he knew I would have a good, long seizure. When I woke up I had a headache, double vision, and stiffness. I took a short nap—feel better now. It was not so easy this time. No PSAS, and that is the point.

4/5/05
I feel indebted to Dr. K for giving me this time free of PSAS—in a way he had to talk me into it.

4/22/05
Dr. G reached out from Boston and helped me find the courage to stay in the world long enough for Dr. K to make me better. I really had plans—it was a close call. I am very grateful to be living, and it is because of my doctors. There are some things beyond the power of words to say.

4/28//05
Looking forward to tomorrow's ECT. Better living through seizures. I really will be fine by tomorrow afternoon.

4/29/05
Dr. K is concerned about my mood, so he started me on a low dose anti-depressant.

5/6/05
Dr. K wants to prolong the time between ECT's and finally stop them. I am worried he is being too optimistic because when it relapses, it is just as awful as ever.

5/7/05
I can't make my next scheduled appointment, so Dr. K wants me to come in 2 days early. It is really too soon, but he is very concerned about me committing suicide if I relapse. He has a right to be—Pennsylvania is full of guns. I have told him about my commitment to my family, but I don't think he's convinced yet. Hope makes all the difference. Why would I kill myself now? Now I know I can be rid of that throbbing basketball between my legs with one maintenance treatment.

5/10/05
The new anti-depressant has lessened the PSAS symptoms and helped normalize our sex life. After all the different therapies, this combination works the best.

5/19/05
Dr. K has agreed to let me prolong the intervals between treatments. He is convinced at last I am stable, which I am.

5/20/05
My girls came by today. They both commented on the weight I have lost—I'm not finished. But absolutely everything is better now. It is glaringly obvious. God bless Dr. K!

6/2/05
I am so grateful to still be here and able to get back to work. Dreadful to think about what I might have done.

6/27/05
Sex with Paul 3 times a week on average is now enough to provide me relief. Paul is also much happier with our love life. He no longer feels he has to try to last forever for my sake. In the beginning, he felt guilty because he couldn't help me enough. I am a happy woman now.

6/28/05
I realized today that the spontaneous orgasms are gone along with the rest of the PSAS symptoms.

7/29/05
I feel like I'm doing extremely well. Despite PSAS relapse at 4 weeks to the day, depression stayed away till treatment at 5 weeks, so I asked to go 6 weeks for treatment, which was just what Dr. K recommended anyway. I am having no obvious side effects and having no trouble keeping up with work at home and at the office. My family says I am better than I ever was.

7/30/05
Dr. K says I am atypical because I wake up from the ECT totally alert and with it. He fears permanent memory loss as a possible long-term side effect, but I'm not having any—not any.

8/01/05
A member of the PSAS online support group who is planning to go to Dr. K for ECT treatment contacted me today.

8/17/05
Marie just e-mailed that after her third ECT, her PSAS seems to be gone. I'm happy for her.

8/22/05
Between times, I forget just how hard it is to carry on. Next ECT is Sept 2. Will be a long 11 days, but who's counting?

8/24/05
Dr. K and I each wanted to stretch the time between the ECT's for our own reasons. I think he is trying to avoid side effects—memory impairment—that I still don't think I am having at this point. I want as long as possible between treatments for my own convenience. I can tolerate the symptoms knowing that this will end on Sept 2. A different matter when it stretched on indefinitely for decades in the future. I would love to never need another ECT. Three days longer between treatments *is* progress. I hesitate to write this or even think it, but the PSAS seems less ferocious when it recurs, making it easier to ignore. I feel like we're finally on the right track.

8/24/06
I can't believe I can now go 14 weeks between treatments. The joy is back in our love life. It has spilled over into our family life. This I can live with.

To learn more about how anti-depressants, menopause, and persistent genital arousal disorder (the contemporary medical term for PSAS) can affect sexual health and the therapies prescribed for Olivia, refer to Part II: The Science.

Marie's Story

I was not able to continue the charade of living in a real hell and getting no medical help for the misery.

Marie's Story

Marie, like Olivia, suffered from persistent sexual arousal syndrome, now called persistent genital arousal disorder. Communicating with other PSAS sufferers on the Internet became Marie's lifeline and a way to find resources to deal with her personal distress.

"I can't be the only one with this problem," I cried, but no one knew how to help me.

My sex life had always been wonderful. My long-term boyfriend had had a very high libido, and I was multi-orgasmic, although always from clitoral orgasms. At forty, I met my very shy and proper, handsome husband. Although we had sex on each date, I was the one to initiate it. Intercourse was over when he reached orgasm. He was unresponsive to my physical needs and uncomfortable with discussing sex, so I made the conscious decision seven years into our marriage that I was no longer going to have sex with him.

Within a few years, I became very depressed. In addition to my ongoing health problems with Tourette's syndrome, my mother was dying from a prolonged illness. Four years after her death, my depression had become severe. I was popping so many different pills, I wasn't able to take proper care of my children or myself, and I wound up being hospitalized for ten days. Over the course of the next year, I was institutionalized on and off four more times. By then, I had put on fifty pounds, and having always been conscious of my weight, I decided that the only way to lose it, against the advice of my doctor, was to go off all my medications, including anti-depressants, cold turkey. Almost three weeks to the day, my world returned from black and white to color. It wasn't long until I had lost the fifty pounds and remained in relatively good health for three months.

Then my life changed—irreversibly it seems—and not just from menopause. I was feeling an intense kind of physical arousal, both very distracting and unrelenting. I had no libido—just a physical need. I tried to have an orgasm to provide some relief to my engorged genital and anal regions, but I couldn't. To make matters worse, I developed a rash over my entire body, including my genitals. The dermatologist who examined me diagnosed it as stress-related psoriasis. I went to my gynecologist out of frustration, but she didn't know what to do to help me. I returned home and masturbated, sweating, for three hours, but couldn't achieve orgasm. I was desperate. I tried looking for answers on the Internet but couldn't find anything. On my next regular appointment with my neurologist for my Tourette's, I brought up my sexual concerns, and he recommended a sexual medicine physician.

I went to the sexual medicine specialist and finally got a diagnosis—PSAS—persistent sexual arousal syndrome. The doctor did not know the cause or the cure for my PSAS, but I finally had the correct words to look up on the Internet. What I found was an online discussion group of women with the same problem as me!

I read everything I could about PSAS and then returned to my doctors. In the meantime, the constant feelings of arousal from the PSAS were taking over my life. The gynecologist suggested a nerve block, the sexual medicine physician suggested a mild, over the counter anesthetic ointment, but someone on the PSAS board suggested a stronger, topical anesthetic to numb the affected region. Someone else suggested freezing water in a condom and placing it over my genitals inside my underwear. I was so grateful to have the suggestions for treatment and someone to talk to.

Even when I was able to have an orgasm, it didn't seem to take anything away other than some of the terrible pressure that kept building and building. I had ordered the topical anesthetic that got me through the PSAS from a compound pharmacy, but the gel was so strong it was causing blisters. After a year of self-treatment, I went to see a doctor who had written a paper on different etiologies of PSAS. He said my blood tests were normal and gave me a list of fourteen things to try and a prescription for a narcotic, as a last resort, for the horrible discomfort that would never leave me. I was becoming suicidal.

Since it had been so difficult for my family during my previous bout with depression, I decided to make every effort to disguise this terrible condition and hide my distress this time. On the surface, I appeared "well" for my husband and boys. Internally, however, I was extremely distraught by the PSAS, so I continued to write to members of the online board. I participated in a survey that revealed that many of the women were in their fifties, and many had started to experience PSAS shortly after suddenly stopping SSRI anti-depressants—just like me. This was one of the medications I had stopped cold turkey. Armed with this information, I decided to contact one of the doctors I had read about on the board, and he was wonderful. He told me about Olivia, with her permission of course, and her successful treatment for PSAS. He introduced us online, but it was a special moment when I met her in person. It was so wonderful to have not only the support of a sexual medicine physician who was knowledgeable and compassionate, but also of a woman who was in my shoes and could totally understand what I was feeling, both physically and mentally. She confided in me that she suffered from depression, and that she had become suicidal after the start of her PSAS symptoms. I confided to her that I, too, felt that way sometimes.

Olivia had found a real solution for her PSAS and was feeling good much of the time. She was even able to work again. I only hoped that there would be help for me. I was not able to continue the charade of living in a real hell and getting no medical help for the misery.

So following Olivia's footsteps and under the care of the same doctors, I proceeded to undergo electroconvulsive therapy that alleviated most of my PSAS symptoms and helped with my depression. I don't remember the emotion of waking up from the third treatment and realizing the PSAS was totally gone. Unfortunately, it didn't remain that way—about twenty percent returned along with psoriasis in the vulvar region. I controlled the psoriasis with a prescription corticosteroid and used maximum strength over the counter medication for the PSAS; I was living relatively pain free. It seems that the stress causing the psoriasis may somehow be related to the PSAS. Most of the arousal I was experiencing was centered in the clitoral area and not my entire genital and anal regions. I used a small vibrator to help me have orgasms to provide needed relief.

I continued to have ECT's using the same protocol as Olivia, but stopped them when they no longer helped. The memory loss was significant and affected my relationship with my family. Now I do my best to control my PSAS with the ice condoms and continue to speak with Olivia for support.

There is no cure for PSAS yet, but it is a blessing to be able to maintain some control over the symptoms.

Olivia and my caring physicians taught me not to give up. A woman does not just have to accept what is happening to her body. Do the research, maintain a positive attitude, and learn from others. Be responsible for yourself—don't become a victim. I refused to!

To learn more about how menopause and persistent genital arousal disorder (the contemporary medical term for PSAS) can affect sexual health and the therapies prescribed for Marie, refer to Part II: The Science.

Leanne's Story

I don't know what upset me more, my lack of desire or my extreme discomfort during sex …

Leanne's Story

Leanne was happily married to a younger man and ready for sex as often as he was, until she reached forty-six. Her healthcare choices regarding her fibroid treatment were based on her desire to maintain a healthy sex life.

My joints were stiff. I could barely walk up the stairs. I was uncomfortable in my own skin. Heart palpitations would start; my legs would get restless. I had trouble sleeping and would kick off the blanket and then freeze when my body temperature returned to normal. My husband called me "Snappy" because I would snap at him all day.

I didn't cry a lot, but I *wanted* to cry *all* the time. I felt like nobody at work understood what I was going through. I was barely functioning—I could hardly lift my arms, and doing that was critical for my job. I had reached the change of life, and my body was reacting like crazy. The hot flashes were unbearable and came like clockwork, almost every thirty minutes. Even more distressing was what had happened to my sex life. For twenty-three years of marriage sex had been great. Since reaching menopause, every time we had intercourse I was in excruciating pain. Ben could barely enter, and the pain didn't subside until he got out.

I first tried over the counter medications and nutritional supplements—didn't help. I would rather be on hormones than live like this, so my gynecologist started me on estrogens despite the negative publicity.

After starting estrogen therapy, the pain during sex disappeared but I started to have severe bleeding. My gynecologist examined me and found a fibroid the size of a golf ball. She recommended a hysterectomy as the only solution and suggested I have my ovaries removed at the same time, since I was past childbearing age. Ironically, one of my customers, a sexual medicine physician, had recently talked to me about his work including the possible effect of hysterectomy on orgasm. I vividly remembered the conversation because my sex life was so important to me—too important to put in jeopardy.

I started searching on the Internet for alternative solutions to hysterectomy and learned about myomectomy. This is a procedure in which fibroid tumors on or near the lining of the uterus can be removed through the cervix. I was fortunate to find a local surgeon who was trained in the myomectomy procedure. If he thought I was a candidate for this surgery, I would be able to keep my uterus. So I returned to my gynecologist to ask her opinion about a myomectomy. She stuck with her original recommendation that I had to have my uterus and ovaries removed. She argued, "You may die of ovarian cancer. Why do you want to keep your ovaries?" I later found out that her fear of my having a myomectomy was because, during her residency training, she had seen a patient die after this procedure.

Despite the hesitancy of my gynecologist who I trusted, I decided to have the myomectomy. The surgeon required that I discontinue the estrogen therapy one month before the procedure. When I stopped the estrogen, my sex life again went "down the tubes," and the debilitating hot flashes returned. I foolishly presumed everything would go back to normal when I started taking the estrogen again after the surgery. Two weeks after the myomectomy, we tried to have sex. I don't know what upset me more, my lack of desire or my extreme discomfort during sex, but I decided it was time to ask my physician customer to take over my sexual healthcare.

The first thing my sexual medicine physician asked me to do was to go to a local blood lab for some tests he prescribed. Evidently, these are not commonly requested tests, because when I went, the lab technician didn't know what tubes to use. When the test results came back, my sexual medicine doctor explained to me that my sex hormone binding globulin was high and my estradiol and unbound testosterone were low. He said that whatever testosterone was there was being attached to the sex hormone binding globulin, leaving little available to work elsewhere in my body, thus impacting my health including my sexual functioning. The doctor explained that having gone on the birth control pill at eighteen for nine years might have affected my sex hormone binding globulin levels. I was lucky that taking the pill had not significantly affected my sex life when I was younger, but I seemed to be paying the price now. I needed to increase my unbound testosterone and decrease my sex hormone binding globulin if I wanted to maintain my overall health and wellbeing.

I was supposed to start with androgen and estrogen therapy. It was frustrating because I wanted to be intimate with my husband, but I was petrified of breast cancer, worried about using testosterone, and not comfortable taking dehydroepiandrosterone. When the doctor explained how to use the different medicines, I thought the treatments sounded like "voodoo." Putting gel on the back of my leg, plus estrogen in my vagina, on my clitoris, in a patch? And taking progesterone because I still had my uterus? But I couldn't live with the hot flashes and my lousy sex life, and I really trusted my sexual medicine physician.

He had me talk to a patient who was successfully using these treatments, which put my mind at ease. So I started the medications.

My sex life returned and the hot flashes went away about the same time. Now the aches and pains are gone, and I can't wait for Ben to come home each evening. I'm totally back to feeling relaxed, in the mood, and ready to experiment sexually. I continue to have blood work done every three months so my doctor can monitor my hormone levels. I remain, however, a prisoner of high sex hormone binding globulin, presumably a result of long-term use of the birth control pill.

Going through menopause has been physically and mentally trying, and I am thankful I didn't have to have a hysterectomy. Now I have a sense of wellbeing and balance. I can keep up with the younger man I married, and I feel really good. "Snappy" has gone!

To learn more about how hysterectomy, menopause, and oral contraception can affect sexual health and the therapies prescribed for Leanne, refer to Part II: The Science.

Debra's Story

I had gotten to the point where I would do anything to avoid sex.

Debra's Story

Debra is a woman in her thirties with young children and pain so severe she was unable to look after them. Married to a man of few words, their communication dwindled because their relationship was more physical than verbal.

Pain! I was in constant pain! The pain was so excruciating, if I was up for the morning with my children, I needed to spend the rest of the day on the couch. I just couldn't move around very much. On the days I went grocery shopping, I couldn't make dinner. If I played with my children that's *all* I could do. I couldn't wear clothing that was tight against my abdomen or touched my genitals, so I lived in loose sweatpants without underwear. Not only did I feel miserable, I looked miserable. Every day was a struggle for me not to become depressed, since my children needed a mother. Looking back, I realize that I was almost totally disabled by the pain.

The pain first started when my two children were toddlers. It began with bladder spasms when I went to bed and sharp pains during intercourse. Since sex had always been central to our relationship, this was very distressing. Although the pain wasn't bad enough at that time to stop us from trying to have sex, my husband knew when things would hurt, and he would stop. Sex wasn't a big deal for *me* anyway because I was exhausted and had lost interest, but I did my best to maintain some kind of a physical relationship for my husband's sake.

I tried to push the pain out of my mind, but the bladder spasms forced me to go to my primary care physician. He sent me to a gynecologist because he suspected a cyst on my ovary. The gynecologist believed the problem would resolve itself, but the bladder pain continued to worsen, so he referred me to a urologist. Despite going through a battery of tests, the urologist was unable to find a reason for the pain. She then referred me to a sexual medicine physician. It was a three-month wait for an appointment, but I had no choice.

The pain, originally triggered by intercourse, was now not only more intense but constant. Depression became overwhelming. My house was a mess, my kids were unhappy that I couldn't play with them, and my husband and I were growing more distant every day. I had sex only to please Pat, but eight months after the start of the pain, we almost had to stop having sex altogether. When I felt good enough to have intercourse, it caused a stabbing pain, and then I lay on the couch for the next three days with throbbing pain. I had gotten to the point where I would do *anything* to avoid sex.

We didn't have any real discussion about what was happening, but my husband has never been a talker. He never gave me a hard time about not having sex, but at the same time there was a lot of tension when he needed to have regular relations. We were both avoiding the problem, which caused stress in all aspects of our relationship. And then one evening, Pat didn't come straight home—he went out for a beer after work. He started going out close to every day and getting really drunk a couple of times, so drunk that he could barely walk straight. I asked a friend of my husband's to talk to him about the drinking and driving. He preferred not to get involved. It got really bad. Caused a lot of problems. I didn't want him around the kids when he was like that, and that issue created even more of a strain on our relationship.

When you are in pain and have lost your desire for sex, you feel guilt as well as discomfort. I don't think that Pat blamed me for avoiding sex, but he was frustrated. I believe that if he had found someone else, he probably would have cheated on me, but I doubt he did, since he was watching a lot of porn. I felt I wasn't being a complete wife. My life was spiraling downward—my health was deteriorating, I couldn't care for my kids, and I was losing my relationship with my husband. It was an extremely stressful time.

I don't know if I can portray how awful it is when you are at your wit's end. I coped by just focusing on my kids. I tried to have fun with them, but it was exhausting. I put myself last. I tried not to think about what was happening. I couldn't talk to anyone about my health because I didn't want anyone to know what I was going through; that's just how I am. No one would have understood anyway, and my husband didn't care. I only told my mother about my pain so she would watch my children when I went to the doctor.

I was very nervous going to see the sexual medicine specialist, and I desperately hoped that he could help me. It is very scary when you've had all the tests and still no one has a solution. Did I have some kind of cancer? Did I have something like MS? This doctor was my last hope. When I went in to see him, he listened to me for as long as I needed to talk. He asked about my pain, and I told him that on a scale of one to ten, pain during the day was a six, but during intercourse it was a nine and stayed at about eight or nine for the next three days. He just sat there and listened and I was *so* grateful. When he examined me, he immediately knew what was wrong with me. I had vestibular adenitis, and it was treatable. If the medical treatments didn't work there was always surgery.

I was so relieved to hear those words that I started crying. He prescribed blood tests to assess my hormone levels, to determine the reason for my lack of desire, and a topical painkiller for the vestibular area, to help me temporarily cope.

My pain had started in August, and my surgery was the following July because the medical treatments were not effective. I was relieved to have the surgery. With four inflamed glands removed, the bladder spasms stopped, and within a day my abdomen relaxed. It had been difficult for me pinpoint the exact locations of the pain before my surgery because I had pain all over. I felt so much better after the surgery, although I continued needing topical pain medication.

Three months later I went back to the specialist. I told him our sex life had returned to normal a few weeks after surgery because I could have sex without pain, so it was time to deal with my desire problems. Fortunately, my arousal response was normal. The doctor prescribed an additional androgen to improve my sexual desire. I applied a small amount of testosterone gel to the back of my legs every day, but I had to remember not to shave around the same time.

We had intercourse about twice a week, and the testosterone gel seemed to help with my desire. However, about five months after the surgery, I started having pain again in the same locations. It was the identical kind of pain as before, although not as severe. Pat was angry when it started again, but at least he wasn't going out drinking any more. He complained, "I thought you were all fixed up." My husband isn't a super supportive person, but that's just the way he is.

I had my second surgery about eight months after the first. The doctor removed more glands. Fortunately, it was an easy recovery, and I started physical therapy soon after. The therapist used biofeedback to help me learn to relax my muscles, and the pain diminished significantly. Then I rented a biofeedback machine to use at home, and exercised every day for twenty minutes. She taught me how to do Kegel exercises for my internal vaginal muscles much more effectively, so that I got stronger doing fewer of them. She worked on my abdominal muscles, stretched out tight muscles, and showed me how to get all my muscles to work together. I was very fortunate to have gone to a physical therapist specializing in women's health so that I could be sexually active again in about two months.

It would have been nice if Pat had been more supportive, but at least we are communicating better now. As I started improving, I saw Pat's behavior change. I don't know what turned him around; maybe he finally realized what was going on. I have always been very attracted to my husband, but with all the stress we were under, I think we would have been divorced if we didn't have kids. Now, we have a more normal relationship, where before we were constantly fighting. I actually initiate sex about a third of the time. Not only is our sex life better, but I'm also feeling better and looking forward to being active with my family once again.

To learn more about how vulvodynia can affect sexual health and the therapies prescribed for Debra, refer to Part II: The Science.

Irene and Harold's Story

Walking had become uncomfortable and she experienced pain in her vagina constantly. Sex was the last thing on her mind.

Irene and Harold's Story

Sexual dysfunction is a couple's issue. This is the story of a husband and wife in a long-term relationship in which each of the partners had to do deal with sexual problems.

The Couple
Irene and Harold have been married for almost fifty years. For the first fifteen years of their marriage, they were both content with their sex life, although Irene found it easier to reach orgasm with masturbation. In her late thirties, she started having problems with pain during intercourse because of vaginal dryness. Since her gynecologist never asked about her sex life, she was hesitant to bring it up. Irene assumed this was a natural part of aging and self-treated, using lubricants to help with the vaginal dryness.

Irene
At forty-one, Irene started experiencing break-through bleeding and was diagnosed with fibroids. That July, just before leaving for vacation, she was given an injection of progesterone that would be effective for three months. Unfortunately, her body overreacted to the drug, and she spent the whole trip crying. Irene's fibroids continued to grow until she looked like she was four months pregnant. Walking had become uncomfortable, and she experienced pain in her vagina constantly. Her doctor started her on the highest dose of combined synthetic estrogen and progesterone hoping the fibroid would shrink. She continued successfully on this hormone regimen for eight years, until forced to stop when she started to lactate from one of her breasts. Without the medication, the pain returned. Irene went from doctor to doctor looking for a solution. She was repeatedly told surgery was now her only option, so at the age of fifty she underwent a hysterectomy and oophorectomy.

The Couple
When Irene was not feeling well, sex was the last thing on her mind. Harold missed having regular intercourse. Ironically, he was unaware that his own

sexual function was diminishing as a result of his acquiring type 2 diabetes. Now, after surgery, Irene was looking forward to resuming their sex life, so she encouraged Harold to seek treatment for his impotence. She knew he would feel better about himself if he could maintain an erection. They went to a sex therapist, and during the conversation, Irene disclosed that in all the years of sexual activity, she had reached orgasm only three times with intercourse. She was hoping the therapist would help Harold overcome his impotence and become a better lover. The therapist called Irene a "spoiled brat" because she wasn't content just to cuddle, so Irene walked out of the session, later encouraging Harold to seek medical treatment for his erectile dysfunction.

Harold

The first doctor Harold went to prescribed testosterone shots for a short period of time, but the therapy didn't solve the problem completely. He went from urologist to urologist looking for a cure, and eventually was prescribed the first oral phosphodiesterase type 5 inhibitor that had just become available. Unfortunately, over time, the medication stopped working. He tried intraurethral insertion, but that proved ineffective for him. Then he participated in a clinical trial for diabetic men using a new PDE5 inhibitor. Harold was having good luck with the trial drug and was able to have successful intercourse again.

Irene

Unfortunately, Irene was "dry as a bone" after her hysterectomy. She wanted to have sex, but intercourse was painful. She had recurrent bacterial infections in her vagina. She went from gynecologist to gynecologist and finally found out that the pH of her vagina was out of balance, that it was too alkaline. The painful infection lasted for three months, making it uncomfortable for Irene to walk or sit.

The Couple

Harold was distressed by the fact that sex really hurt Irene. He suggested she go to his sexual medicine physician because Harold had seen women patients in the office. Weeks went by before she agreed, but when the pain became so bad during intercourse that Irene was desperate, she decided to go with her husband. She was fascinated that Harold was going, and that he was so hopeful about his treatment. She was told she would meet with the psychologist, as well as the doctor, and assumed she would need to go to sex therapy. Maybe they just weren't doing it right!

Irene

She had seen a sex therapist before, but it was for Harold's impotence. It was liberating for Irene to be able to discuss her own issues with the psychologist. She also completed the Female Sexual Function Index, a questionnaire to determine whether or not a woman has sexual dysfunction. Then Irene saw Harold's doctor, and he told her he could help. He looked at the lab results she had brought with her, and saw Irene's testosterone and dehydroepiandrosterone values were practically non-existent. The doctor did a physical exam, including the Q-tip test and a blood flow test. That felt weird to her, but Irene knew her husband trusted this physician. The doctor thought he knew the problem, she had developed vulvar vestibulitis syndrome after her hysterectomy and oophorectomy, so he sent Irene home with the prescriptions she needed.

The Couple

In about a month, Irene started to feel better. Her concentration and energy had improved, and she was interested in having sex again. The pain during intercourse had lessened significantly, and virtually disappeared by using a lubricant. But there was still something wrong. Irene and Harold had been through so much for so long with each of their sexual health issues, they decided they needed to go back to the psychologist for a few sex therapy sessions. The therapist focused on improving the couple's communication and relaxation skills, using behavioral methodology to encourage relaxation for sex. He suggested that using a vibrator would help Irene to have orgasms, because finger manipulation no longer worked. Irene and Harold continued to see the therapist weekly for three months.

Their sex life was once again disrupted when the clinical trial for diabetics was over, and Harold's access to the medication stopped. The couple didn't know how many years it would be before this new drug would be available by prescription, so they were forced to consider alternative therapies. They had gone too far to quit now. Irene accompanied Harold when he returned to the sexual medicine physician's office, where she was taught to inject medicine into Harold's penis so he could maintain an erection. This therapy was initially successful, but eventually Harold developed Peyronie's disease, scarring which caused a bend in the penis. This made intercourse very painful for Irene, so they just stopped having sex. Irene was being treated for her sexual dysfunction, feeling better about herself and now, once again, Harold could not function. After a lot of discussion, they decided that the only answer was for Harold to get a penile implant. In the meantime, the doctor suggested that Irene use a small vibrator with lubrication, then progress to a larger one, to prepare for being sexually active and intimate again.

Irene

After Harold's implant, the couple believed they had found their solution. Irene, however, kept getting yeast infections right after sex. She was having problems with her clitoris, which had become so ultra-sensitive, it could only be touched in a certain way. She felt like she had a diaper rash on her clitoris. The physician suggested removing the hood of the clitoris to allow the yeast infection under the hood to be treated, but for the time being local anti-fungal agents managed the infection. Eventually, however, the hood would have to be removed.

The Couple

Now, in their late sixties, the couple is enjoying a healthy sex life once again. Irene has had her sexual health issues, Harold his, but their sexual health concerns were a shared problem, and their treatments, a shared solution. They have talked freely with their children, telling them about Harold's implant and Irene's treatment. They want their children to know that maintaining sexual intimacy is an important aspect of a relationship, no matter what your age.

To learn more about how hysterectomy, male partner's sexual health, and menopause can affect sexual health and the therapies prescribed for Irene, refer to Part II: The Science.

Elaine's Interview

I felt like my whole life had changed—I became severely depressed. I was avoiding sex because of intense pain and not for lack of interest.

Elaine's Interview

Elaine is a thirty-nine-year-old woman whose sexual function was impacted by prolonged and debilitating pain. Her interview was so compelling that we chose to share some quotations taken directly from it.

Unless you have been in chronic pain, you have no idea how profoundly this affects all aspects of your life.

We managed to have sex three or four times a week until the pain became unbearable. Although I hate doctors, this forced me to go to my gynecologist for help. I told my gynecologist that if he didn't do something, I would kill myself because I knew I couldn't live with the pain.

I went to doctor after doctor, but no one made any suggestions for pain management.

I felt like my whole life had changed—I became severely depressed. I was avoiding sex because of intense pain and not for lack of interest.

The pain was so debilitating, I could barely get out of bed.

I learned there was a thin line between pleasure and pain. I would wake in the middle of the night in such excruciating pain that I would ask if we could have sex, hoping it would give me some relief. I would do anything to take the pain away and be a wife and mother again.

I was desperate for a solution. I was referred to a sexual medicine specialist and counted the days until I could see him.

He knew exactly what it was. The hood was completely covering my clitoris, causing this awful, awful pain. It compounded a yeast infection under the hood of my clitoris.

I started conservative therapy with an anti-fungal cream. It helped by treating the yeast infection under the hood of the clitoris, stopping the extreme pain, and the need to have orgasm all the time to provide relief.

I still had the bad burning and stinging, but the doctor said the medication was definitely working and to continue using it.

I needed to be on pain medication or have my clitoris removed. The prescription made the pain tolerable, but whenever I tried to stop the medication, the pain would get ahead of me.

The anti-fungal medication wasn't working any more. I had surgery to remove the hood of the clitoris, believing that it would solve my problems. I felt good for one week.

At my post-op check up, there was a little redness on my clitoris, so I was sent to a genital dermatologist. I was put on heavy doses of an oral pain medicine, normally used to control seizures, and warned that it might take two to three years before I felt better. I thought, "This medication can't be good for me."

The treatment didn't stop the pain because it wasn't neurologic. I was started on an ultra-potent steroid cream for dermatitis of the frenulum instead. The pain from the surgery finally subsided. The irritation also seemed to disappear, so I stopped using the anti-fungal medication.

I was feeling better, so I started exercising again—I was getting my life back. I wasn't interested in sex, but I had intercourse every couple of weeks anyway. I could reach orgasm, but it was easier for me to masturbate. Some areas around my clitoris were just too sensitive to leave to my husband's touch.

I still had genital burning and stinging, even though I used the steroid cream regularly. I was referred to a pain management clinic, where I was prescribed a pain patch.

Removing the hood of the clitoris cleared the original irritation there, so I was convinced that getting air to this sensitive area would cure the problem. Then I remembered that my doctor had mentioned that my labia were unusually long, in comparison to the women whose surgery had been successful. I decided to have labial reduction surgery, because where the labia overlapped, the yeast continued to grow.

My labia were reduced from four and a half centimeters to one centimeter. This wasn't the time to be conservative—I didn't want to have a third surgery.

I feel such a sense of relief that the irritation has healed, the burning has disappeared, and the pain is under control.

To protect my health, I have changed my diet, and when I exercise, I shower carefully immediately after to avoid getting another yeast infection. I have a life again after this two-year ordeal. Despite the strain on our relationship and the frustration of the ongoing pain, my husband and I are still happily married.

To learn more about how metabolic syndrome and vulvodynia can affect sexual health and the therapies prescribed for Elaine, refer to Part II: The Science.

Thea's Thoughts

He was the first person who really talked to me about my sexual health issues, and all my pent up frustration and emotion came out.

Thea's Thoughts

Thea's relationship with her husband was deteriorating due to her lack of libido. She assumed her loss of interest in sex was the result of early menopause, but sought help because of the detrimental impact it was having on her marriage.

I can't even remember when it actually happened. I do know, however, it didn't happen overnight … it was gradual. I probably wouldn't have realized it if my husband hadn't pointed it out, and continued to point it out, over, and over, and over. I just didn't want to have sex. I avoided it … I was actively avoiding it. I avoided anything that would stimulate him because that could lead to sex. I made sure that he didn't see me naked. I let him touch me, but I didn't let him caress me. I would push him away. Over time, I became distressed because I loved my husband and used to enjoy sex too.

I am forty-nine now, and the problem started in my early forties. Eight years ago, I tried to talk to a doctor about this. He basically ignored me. Since I was embarrassed to talk about it, I let it go and didn't mention it to another doctor for a few years, until I became desperate when our relationship was breaking down—we were headed for divorce. I went to a new doctor and told him I had no interest in sex. His response was, "Don't worry about it. You have a very stressful job. You just need to make time for sex." This was not the solution, and fights about sex escalated. We were both miserable.

Then one day when I turned on CNN, a sexual medicine physician, Dr. Irwin Goldstein, was being interviewed about biologic causes of women's sexual dysfunction. As I watched him, I realized he was describing *me*, and I was in shock. I couldn't believe that somebody actually understood my problems. Listening to him inspired me to return to my gynecologist who suggested I probably had psychological problems, and would benefit from seeing a marriage counselor. I *knew* that wasn't it. I went onto the CNN Web site, found Dr. Goldstein's contact information, and called for an appointment.

Despite being happy to have found Dr. Goldstein, I broke down and cried throughout the entire interview with his psychologist. He was the first person who really talked to me about my sexual health issues, and all my pent up frustration and emotion came out. I don't even know where these feelings came from, but it was such a relief to finally be understood.

When I met with Dr. Goldstein, it was obvious that he had treated many women with problems similar to mine. The experience was surreal, the questions he asked … the physical exam … the sensitivity test. I had always assumed that reaching menopause at thirty-nine was the reason I didn't want to have sex in my forties, but Dr. Goldstein believed there were other factors contributing to my sexual dysfunction. He told me his theories about oral contraceptives and biking, each being a potential cause of sexual health problems. I had started taking birth control pills in college, used them forever, and I had been an avid biker, riding fourteen to twenty-one miles a day, four to five days a week, for ten years. I learned I had limited sensation in my vestibule, and that could have been a result of all my biking, however I still needed blood tests. Who knows what my hormone levels would be after being on birth control pills for so long and being post-menopausal. Dr. Goldstein could not give me a definitive diagnosis until he had all the test results.

Three weeks later, I returned with blood tests in hand. Dr. Goldstein explained the significance of the results, and I was ecstatic to have a diagnosis: hypothyroidism and hypogonadism. He referred me to an endocrinologist for management of my hypothyroidism, and prescribed dehydroepiandrosterone, testosterone, and local estrogen for my sexual health. I was beginning to have some burning with intercourse. Dr. Goldstein explained that this was to be expected, because he had found signs of vaginal atrophy during the exam. The medications I was now starting would alleviate these symptoms. In addition to treating me for my sexual dysfunction, Dr. Goldstein gave me medication to manage my genital herpes. As sad as it may seem, when I had monthly breakouts in the past, I was happy because it gave me a "legitimate" reason not to have sex.

For the first three months of treatment, I was excited about sex. I think the medications must have had a placebo effect, because I soon lost my interest again. My sexual medicine physician prescribed more blood tests. Over the course of the next two years, he suggested several different treatments for me to try, including increasing the androgens, but nothing worked. It was really disappointing not to have my drive back, but I no longer avoided sex at all costs. Receptivity to my husband's sexual advances was *definitely* an improvement.

When the doctor started me on a dopamine agonist, things changed for the better. I started to look forward to sex … have thoughts about sex … but the side effects of hair growth and acne from the increasing doses of androgens made me unhappy. I would wake up in the morning and look in the mirror, and think I was getting better, but by mid day I had lumps (not just pimples) on my face. This so distressed me that I contacted both my sexual medicine physician, who adjusted the testosterone dose and prescribed an enzyme inhibitor, and my dermatologist, who prescribed an additional medication. I was relieved when I was finally able to get these side effects under control.

In retrospect, I realize my husband had been serious about a divorce. At the time, he thought I was having an affair, because he couldn't think of any other reason for me not wanting sex. When I started my treatment, he couldn't understand why it didn't always work. Things have gotten better; we don't fight about sex anymore. I only hope that the medications keep working, because I don't want a divorce....

To learn more about how menopause, oral contraception, and thyroid conditions can affect sexual health and the therapies prescribed for Thea, refer to Part II: The Science.

Trisha's Letter

I used to be aroused quickly just like you, and seeing your sexual response is a constant reminder to me of my own inadequacy.

Trisha's Letter

Trisha is a peri-menopausal woman concerned about the future of her relationship because of her sexual health issues. Confused and vulnerable, she wanted to get better for her lover, as well as for herself.

Dear Bobbie,

I want you to know how much I love you. I don't mean to keep hurting you this way, yet I find myself apologizing, once again, for rolling over and going to sleep. This has been happening a lot lately, and I know this distresses you. I used to look forward to going to bed, and what would happen next, and now I don't even care. I've totally lost interest in sex, but I am telling you from my heart that you are still the person I want to spend the rest of my life with.

After my break up ten years ago, I became seriously depressed and had to go on medication for a year. I realize now that it was during that terrible period in my life that I lost my desire for sex. I was so distraught that I had no interest in even having a relationship until I met you. Every time I was with you, I was so turned on that I couldn't wait to have sex with you. It felt good to enjoy sex again, like I did in my 20's and 30's, and I was convinced that my past sexual problems were finally gone.

It is difficult for me to even write these words but the reality is that even though I recovered emotionally from the breakup, I never really recovered my sex drive or desire for sex. In retrospect, I can only presume that the great sex we had when we first met was due to the newness of our relationship.

Now, when you and I kiss, you are immediately turned on. I used to be aroused quickly just like you, and seeing your sexual response is a constant reminder to me of my own inadequacy. Please don't think that I am rejecting you, I love you, and I love being touched by you, but I miss my sexual response ... the heavy breathing, and feeling my genitals tingle. I feel badly because we don't make love as often as you want.

We've become more like best friends and companions than lovers. I know that makes you unhappy—it makes me unhappy too.

Because I love you so much, I know my problems must be physical and not due to trouble in our relationship. I've tried to talk with my gynecologist, and he gave me pamphlets on menopause to read, but didn't really have a solution. He assumed that because I am now in my 40's, my problem was from peri-menopause, but I had these issues long before. There is something wrong with my body, and I don't know what to do.

I worry about our future together. I am so afraid my sexual issues are undermining our stability and security as a couple. You tell me that all the time. I pray I won't lose you over this issue, but I know in my heart that you are a beautiful, sexual being who wants and needs intimacy. I desperately want and need to be the one to provide it for you.

I acknowledge that this is my problem, and I feel guilty that I haven't worked hard enough to treat it. I've tried to find a resolution myself, and I'm not sure I have the energy to try again. I convinced my gynecologist to give me a medication that I had read about, and I used it on three separate occasions, but I panicked when I started getting acne. I realize that you probably think I'm not committed to getting better, but my deepest fear is that I will try the treatment again and still won't return to normal. Then, what will happen to us?

It's easier for me to be affectionate and non-sexual, but that is so common among us lesbians. I know that as weeks pass, and we haven't made love, you get frustrated and angry and feel hopeless about the situation, believing that there is something missing in our relationship, which I know there is. We are getting along so well in every other way—I want to get better for you as well as for me. I promise, I will find a doctor who specializes in sexual medicine, and I will do whatever he tells me.

Please, be patient with me. I love you, and I don't want to lose you.

Trisha

To learn more about how anti-depressants can affect sexual health and the therapies available to Trisha, refer to Part II: The Science.

Tracey's Story

When Tracey attended the conference, she wasn't too distressed with what she learned, until she went to a breakout session on surgical menopause.

Tracey's Story

After being diagnosed as BRCA positive while still in her thirties, Tracey was forced to examine what lay ahead. Fortunately, she and her husband were able to make the difficult decisions together.

"Tracey, it's your cousin Ellie. I have bad news. I've been diagnosed with cancer in the other breast. I can't believe I have to go through all of this again. They need to operate as soon as possible. My doctor thinks I probably have a mutation of the BRCA gene. Have you ever heard of that? You may want to get tested."

In shock, Tracey hung up the phone. Everyone thought of her as the "girl next door," with a loving husband, two healthy children, and a happy home. Their lives seemed perfect until Ellie called. Tracey had no idea how life altering this information would be. Her cousin had just been diagnosed with a second primary breast cancer, and she was only thirty-eight. This was a "red flag" that the breast cancer could be genetic.

Her mother, an only child, had been killed in an automobile accident at thirty-six, so Tracey had no idea if there was a history of breast cancer on that side of the family. This cousin was on her father's side. Ellie had been diagnosed with and treated for breast cancer at thirty-four, but that was not considered a risk factor for Tracey. When her cousin developed a new primary cancer in her other breast, the oncologist became concerned about the breast cancer susceptibility gene, BRCA. Tracey decided she needed to know whether she carried a mutation of the BRCA gene. She was thirty-eight and pregnant when she got diagnosed as BRCA positive.

Tracey had some tough decisions to make. She didn't have cancer, but she was at high risk for it, so she opted to go through genetic counseling. BRCA issues are very complex, as there are a variety of choices. Because she wanted to nurse her baby for six months, Tracey knew that she had time before decisions had to be made regarding removal of her breasts and ovaries.

Standard treatment for a BRCA positive patient is to remove the breasts and ovaries even though there is no cancer present. There is a strong association between ovarian cancer, as well as breast cancer, with the BRCA mutation. With ovarian cancer, there are no options—ovaries are removed after the woman completes child bearing or turns forty.

Tracey was stunned, because the discussions with her physicians about her options were so casual. She knew she had to have her ovaries removed because of the risk of ovarian cancer, but there was limited information from her doctors about what would happen to her as a result of the surgery. She was told, however, she would immediately experience surgical menopause with all the accompanying side effects. When Tracey pressed the doctors for more information, they reassured her that they would treat each problem as it occurred. Because she had a wonderful relationship with her husband, Tracey was particularly anxious about her sexual function after the surgery, but was comfortable with her doctors' plans for management. She decided that before making any decisions, she would gather as much information as possible regarding her options. She visited different doctors, searched on the Internet, and found out about a local conference for women with the BRCA mutation.

When Tracey attended the conference, she wasn't too distressed with what she learned, until she went to a breakout session on surgical menopause. The majority of the women in the session were absolutely miserable. They complained that they were depressed, and very unhappy sexually. Surgical menopause had forced the aging process, hitting each woman like a ton of bricks.

Since most of the women at the conference had breast cancer, their alternatives were limited. Many were on anti-depressants or a combination of other medications in an attempt to deal with the symptoms; for most people, these were not effective. Seeing how unhappy they were, Tracey became terrified. "Would this be my story? I'm thirty-eight years old, approaching what should be the peak of my life, and I'm facing removal of my ovaries, and this terrible outcome."

Hormone therapy is controversial for people with this BRCA positive status, and much more controversial for survivors of breast cancer.

Tracey went to several endocrinologists after reading about menopause. She was reassured that since she didn't have breast cancer, hormone therapy would be an option. But they all believed in the approach of dealing with the symptoms as they arose. As one of the doctors said, "You might not have any symptoms. You might sail through."

She kept wondering, even if she didn't have all of those symptoms, would she really want to be without hormones for the next ten years? Even if she felt fine, wasn't there a potential problem here? When Tracey asked her doctor about this, his reply was, "Hormones in and of themselves are more harmful in your situation. We can address the bone loss with medication." Getting increasingly uncomfortable with this response, and more and more concerned, Tracey chose not to return to that doctor.

She met with ten different physicians, all of whom believed that a woman in Tracey's situation needed to have her uterus removed, along with her ovaries, so there would be no need for progesterone. None of these doctors addressed the sexual issues resulting from the surgery despite the published data that hysterectomy could have an impact on sexual functioning. So Tracey met with a sexual medicine physician, who explained the potential impact of a hysterectomy and oophorectomy on her sexual health. They discussed the option of keeping her uterus and just removing her ovaries, so she would be able to maintain her ability to have internal orgasms, an important part of her sexual satisfaction. This would mean that if she used estrogen she would also need to take progesterone. Tracey decided not to have a hysterectomy and take bioidentical estrogen and progesterone. This would also help resolve the vaginal atrophy that the doctor had discovered when he examined her.

> *Although more safety data are needed, by using bioidentical hormones, the doctor could follow Tracey's blood test values closely and keep them in the normal range. If research determined that the progesterone increased cancer risk, she could always have a hysterectomy at a later date.*

Six months after her baby was born, Tracey had her ovaries removed, because she knew they presented a cancer risk. With ovarian cancer, the risk increases forty percent after forty for women who are BRCA positive, so she wanted to do it as soon as she could. Unfortunately, she had a harsh transition after the oophorectomy into menopause. She immediately went on hormone therapy, an estrogen patch and daily progesterone, however Tracey had a terrible reaction to the progesterone. For the first three months on the medication, she was a wreck, weepy, emotional, agitated, and very depressed. She was already anxious about her outcome from the surgery and now Tracey was horrified to realize she had become just like the women she had met at the BRCA conference.

One of Tracey's major concerns had been regarding her sexual response, and she immediately noticed changes after the surgery. "I felt dull, just completely dull. In the past, even if I went through a cycle where I was not interested in sex, I was always very easily aroused and always reached orgasm. It was never a problem." Orgasm was now almost impossible for Tracey. She had some sensation, but it wasn't heightened like before. On occasion, when she was able to achieve orgasm, it was muted—she was very frustrated.

Tracey returned to the sexual medicine physician, and he drew blood for hormone tests. Based on elevated blood levels of progesterone, he lowered her daily dose, and the emotional side effects immediately disappeared. Then, he addressed her sexual issues in consultation with her oncologist. Because he had baseline hormone values from before the surgery, her sexual medicine physician felt comfortable starting appropriate treatment for her sexual dysfunction. Hormone therapy included local estrogens and systemic testosterone gel. Tracey really noticed a difference in sensation. "Although my orgasms were not where they were before in terms of intensity, they were vastly improved. I was interested in sex again, and in about four or five months I finally felt emotionally and physically stable."

The next step was determining whether or not to have a double mastectomy. Having healthy breasts removed is a personal decision, unlike that of the oophorectomy, because breasts can be closely monitored. Consequently, Tracey was having frequent clinical exams and breast screening, alternating mammograms and MRI's, the thought being that the survival rate was high with any breast cancer diagnosed early. But her feeling was that even if the cancer was caught very early, treatment would involve chemotherapy and radiation, and she just didn't want to go there. And she didn't want to be living from test to test.

Tracey's husband actually pushed her quite a bit to do the surgery. He really felt strongly about it … the idea of raising three children on his own terrified him. His mother had died of breast cancer when he was very young, and his brother's wife recently died of breast cancer, leaving behind two small children. His family had obviously been greatly impacted by the disease. This made it a very easy decision, and they never wavered from it.

Having her ovaries removed had been very difficult, but the double mastectomy was nothing. Tracey felt so lucky—she never got a diagnosis of breast cancer. And since she didn't actually have cancer, she was able to have the reconstruction surgery at the time of the mastectomy *and* keep her nipples. Before surgery, nipple sensation was an important part of sexual stimulation for her. This made the surgery a little more complicated, as some residual breast tissue must remain, but it made a difference to her to wake up and have her nipples. This isn't an option for women with cancer.

Tracey missed breast sensation because nipple stimulation always helped her with arousal. "What I have now is prickly, but I have hopes that, as the area heals, this will improve. It was such a big part of my sex life that I feel a great loss." Oral sex became more important for Tracey with the loss of breast tissue.

"It has been a long nine months adjusting to all of this. I give my husband a lot of credit for being so supportive." Over the course of this ordeal, most of the doctors Tracey met discounted the issues of sexual health, because their primary concern was keeping her cancer-free. There are, however, doctors who will be sympathetic and work with a woman regarding her personal concerns. Everyone has options, but you have to find the right doctor. Tracey hoped her actions would prove to be a positive example for her three daughters, but prayed *they* would *never* have to go through this.

To learn more about how cancer treatment can affect sexual health and the therapies prescribed for Tracey, refer to Part II: The Science.

Lil's Story

As my tolerance for sexual activity decreased,
my distress increased.

Lil's Story

Lil, co-author of this book, lost her sexual desire at the age of twenty-nine, after giving birth to her first child. For over a quarter of a century, she went from doctor to doctor seeking a solution. In her fifties, Lil finally found a sexual medicine physician and confirmed what she knew all along: it wasn't "in her head," it was a biologic problem.

Every time I picked up the phone to make the call, my stomach hurt. After twenty-eight years I had found a doctor who *might* be able to help, so why was I so afraid to make the appointment? If I didn't make this call, would I be passing up an opportunity to finally find a solution?

When Wayne and I were first married, we had a great sexual relationship. We didn't talk about sex because it wasn't an issue; it was just something that was spontaneous and fun. At twenty-eight, I became pregnant with our first child. The pregnancy was uneventful, except for losing my desire for sex. During my Lamaze class, the instructors said that this happens to many women, so I didn't worry about it. My daughter's birth was without complications, but my desire for sex did not return. I reasoned it was because I was so focused on the baby's care, and that I hadn't completely recovered. The night before my six-week check-up we had sex, and for the first time in my life, I had difficulty becoming aroused and experienced pain with penetration. When I asked the doctor about this, she told me it was normal after an episiotomy, and it would get better over time.

As the months passed, my interest in sex continued to be non-existent. When we did have sex, I had absolutely no lubrication, making a once pleasurable experience, painful. The baby "loved life," she was awake much of the time, and Wayne and I were constantly exhausted. I convinced myself that when the baby slept through the night, our sex life would return to normal.

In the back of my mind I was worried. What had happened to my body? Did this happen to other women? I needed to know, but former Catholic schoolgirls didn't talk about sex. When I finally found the courage to ask my friends, all young mothers, they claimed their sex lives had returned to normal after each birth.

My lack of desire and lubrication became a source of great anxiety and distress for me. Before I had my daughter, just a kiss from Wayne would arouse me, and now my body wasn't responding at all. Not only was I uninterested, I was so dry that sex had become painful. Here I was at twenty-nine, with a new baby, a sweet, loving husband, and sex had become just another chore on my weekly to do list. How long would I have to wait for my body to recover from childbirth?

At my annual check up, I once again brought up my unresolved sexual issues to my gynecologist, including the fact that I could no longer wear tampons. No matter how heavy my menstrual flow, the tampon felt like sandpaper inside me. When the doctor examined me, she said that everything looked fine, the vaginal walls had normal lubrication, and since my periods were regular, my problem was "not physical." I was convinced there must be other women who felt this way, and if I just found the right physician, everything could be returned to normal.

Two years later, at thirty-three, my son was born. As bizarre as it seems now, I hoped that this birth would reverse the problems—no such luck. I continued to have problems with a lack of desire and lubrication. At the advice of a doctor, I started to use lubricants to help with dryness. The pain lessened, but my interest did not improve. The only time I thought about sex was when my husband brought it up.

Over the next few years, I went to more gynecologists who told me the same thing. Because no doctor could determine a biologic reason, each made the assumption that the problem was psychologic. I can't tell you how many times I heard, "It's probably in your head," "You need to learn to relax," or "Have someone take your kids and go away for the weekend with your husband." Trying to be helpful, one physician told me not to leave his office until I made an appointment with a psychologist. I left his office, crying as I shuffled to the car. I knew my problem was not psychological; that it had to be linked to childbirth. My sexual functioning had turned off, like a switch in my body, and no amount of therapy could change that.

My identity as a woman was gone. I existed from day to day, robotic, doing what needed to be done, taking care of my children, and going to work. I guess it was my survival strategy. My husband and I talked about this issue often, as it upset him greatly. Despite my reassurances to Wayne that it wasn't him, I was filled with conflict and doubt about myself. If I truly loved my husband, why wasn't I interested in having sex with him? But I didn't want to have sex with anyone. I felt like I did when I had been a child; sex just wasn't in my consciousness.

During the next decade, I focused my energy on teaching, raising the children, and attending graduate school. Our sex life was as "normal" as it could be, until my mid-forties when I entered peri-menopause, and my problems worsened. As my tolerance for sexual activity decreased, my distress increased. I can remember starting to cry, when Wayne initiated sex, "I can't do it, just leave me alone." I just didn't want to be touched. We were both miserable, yet I reassured him that I loved him, because I did. Out of desperation, I told my husband to have an affair and not tell me. He was devastated at the suggestion, and I was devastated at the thought.

Wayne had survived a life-threatening illness early in our marriage, and as a result we had a very strong emotional relationship, but our sexual relationship was now based on guilt. He didn't want to pressure or burden me, except when physical need for sex became so intense he would ask, leaving him feeling guilty for asking. And I felt guilty because my body did not respond. I remember often thinking, "Please don't ask me to have sex tonight, I can't. I don't have the patience or the tolerance. I can't dig deep enough in myself anymore to do one more thing."

I went to many doctors, and even though it was embarrassing for me to bring up my sexual health concerns, I never stopped asking. It was extremely discouraging to see the negative reactions of many of those physicians. Clearly, they were uncomfortable when I brought up the topic, although I didn't know whether it was because of their lack of knowledge or their own "issues," but I remained determined to find a solution.

As I approached menopause, we had sexual relations about once a month—out of guilt. I adored my husband, and I wanted him to be happy. Wayne is a very sensitive, perceptive man who couldn't bear putting more pressure on me than I was already experiencing. Although he would have preferred to have sex more frequently, he seemed to accept the way things were. I was the one who couldn't accept it. "I don't know what is wrong with me." I cried with Wayne. I cried by myself. The memory of this time still brings tears to my eyes.

Out of desperation, I took a risk and talked to my friends again about their sex lives, now that we were all peri-menopausal, but they all responded that everything was still fine. One friend said, "Hey, if there's no sex, what is life worth living for? That's what makes life fun." All I could think was, I wonder what it would be like to feel that way … because I didn't.

As I entered menopause, our intimate moments became rare. I seldom let Wayne hug me or even hold my hand because I knew where it might lead, and I couldn't go there. Looking back, I realize how fortunate I was to be married to a man who loved me, no matter what. I wouldn't have blamed him if he had left me. My heart was breaking—he deserved so much more in a relationship.

Wayne never pressured me into seeking help. When Viagra™ came out, I remembered saying to him that maybe, now that they had a drug for men, they would have something to help me—that was my first hope. Soon after, the words "female sexual dysfunction" were used on a TV talk show and in the news. Suddenly, I knew what my problem was. Now, my world began to come into focus. It wasn't just me, and it wasn't "in my head"—I could have a real medical problem. So what was I supposed to do now? I was discouraged and depressed and had lost all confidence in the health care profession. I didn't believe that I would ever find a doctor who could help me with this issue.

One year later, as I transitioned through menopause, I began to suffer from continuous, burning vaginal pain. Nothing gave me relief, and intercourse made it worse. I also began to have constant discharge. When the pain became debilitating, I tried over the counter remedies, but finally gave in and went for a physical. I didn't realize at the time, but this would be a turning point in my quest for a solution.

I was fifty-five years old in 2002, when I met a gynecologist who actually *asked me* if I was satisfied with my sex life. It was such a relief to be asked and know that I didn't have to summon up the courage, once again, to bring up the topic. I told her about my problem, explaining that since my daughter's birth, I had had no interest in sex and had difficulty with lubrication. An advocate of women's healthcare, she told me that if men had a right to a healthy sex life, the same should be true for women. Then, she gave me the name of a local urologist who specialized in sexual medicine. As I walked out the door, she reassured me that I would find a solution … the first encouraging words I had heard in twenty-seven years!

Sexual medicine? I did an Internet search on the physician recommended by my gynecologist. He had published numerous papers on sexual medicine and had a comprehensive Web site to educate his patients, as well as physicians. I began to feel confident that this was a legitimate field. Yet, I was still reluctant, because I didn't know if I was prepared to hear from another doctor that I didn't have a physical problem, when *I knew I did*. It took me six months to make the call.

I worried about what my visit would be like. What kinds of questions would be asked? Would I have the courage to have a conversation about the most intimate details of my life with a stranger, a man? How were sexual health problems diagnosed? What tests were done and medications prescribed? As much as I wanted a resolution, I was terrified, but I believed that I *deserved* a healthy sex life. This issue had created unbelievable tension in our marriage for many years. There was something wrong with me, I was broken—I wasn't normal. That feeling was with me every moment of every day. How wonderful would it be if that terrible feeling of inadequacy were gone?

I knew that if I made the appointment, I would keep it. I vowed to walk through my fears and make the call. For three days I had tried, and now, it was time. I lifted the phone and dialed.

When the day of my appointment finally arrived, I entered the waiting room, extremely anxious but determined. I had to complete patient questionnaires inquiring about my levels of desire, arousal, orgasm, and pain with intercourse, as well as answer questions about my mental health. I met with a psychologist first, and felt remarkably comfortable speaking with him. Although it was a short conversation, it eased some of my anxiety. When I told him about my earlier experience, refusing to go to a psychologist to deal with my sexual issues because I felt the problems were physical, he agreed. That was the first time ever that a healthcare professional openly supported my belief that the problem wasn't "in my head." Then, he brought me to meet the sexual medicine physician.

After the initial interview, the doctor told me that he was pretty sure he knew what my problem was, even before he had all the test results. He also said the most encouraging words that I'd ever heard, "… and I think we have a solution." I was elated. A physician listened to me, had the knowledge to see that my lack of desire and lubrication could have stemmed from a medical problem, and had a solution! After a physical exam and several diagnostic procedures, I learned that I had limited sensation in my vaginal area that could have been a result of nerve damage during childbirth or some other injury. The doctor explained that a lack of sensation would impact my ability to have normal arousal and lubrication. When I heard that, I immediately felt a sense of relief, a sense of validation that at least one of my problems was physical. The doctor gave me a prescription for blood tests and reassured me he was going to help. He would start me on a treatment regimen as soon as he received the results.

I couldn't wait to tell my husband. Picture a fifty-six-year-old woman skipping through a parking garage. Wayne was laughing at me. I got in and screamed in excitement, "I think we found the answer!" We both felt a sense of relief and hope, and at the same time were cautiously optimistic because it *had* been a long time.

I returned to the sexual medicine physician when the blood test results were complete. The diagnosis was obvious: hypogonadism. I had extremely low levels of testosterone and dehydroepiandrosterone, so I was prescribed androgen therapy. Three months later, I repeated the original blood tests and had a follow up visit. Unfortunately, while I had seen an increase in my energy levels and overall sense of wellbeing, there had been little change in desire or arousal. Based on the new blood tests results, my doctor decreased the dehydroepiandrosterone and added testosterone gel to the regimen.

I began to notice a difference in about six weeks. Sex was now in my consciousness. I found myself walking the canned goods aisle of the supermarket, distracted by thoughts of sex. Compared to my levels of desire and arousal before my daughter was born, I was now halfway there. And on retesting, my hormone blood levels had improved. Although there was some minimal hair growth on my face and the application site of the gel, the long-awaited return of my sexual health far outweighed the few trips to my new friend, the electrologist.

Although Wayne and I have always been best friends, our renewed intimacy and closeness had an extremely positive impact on our relationship. There was a whole new dimension of joy to our lives, as we found ourselves laughing and playing more—life no longer seemed so intense and serious. I also began to feel better about myself. For so many years, I had existed with no sense of sexuality, just doing what was necessary to get through my life. My family and friends had no idea of what I had been through or the impact on my self-esteem. They saw me as accomplished and confident. Now I wasn't a fraud; I felt like a woman and enjoyed it. I wanted to express my *new* sense of self with a *new* look and in *new* ways.

I was thrilled about regaining my sexual function, but I still had constant burning around the opening of my vagina. I desired and enjoyed intercourse, but dealt with the constant burning by using topical medication four or five times per day. Evidently, the vestibular glands had become exposed due to years of androgen insufficiency. After a year of attempting to treat the problem with medical therapies, the pain had not resolved, so my doctor suggested surgery.

It is amazing how one can adjust to living with pain, so I thought, "Is it really that bad that I need to have surgery? Maybe I can just cope with this." Then I visualized myself at eighty years old, with arthritic hands, trying to put on the topical medication to dull the pain. Not a realistic option. So after years of seeking a solution and finally finding it, here was another obstacle, and I tried not to be discouraged.

The surgery went well, and I was back home that afternoon. I didn't need the prescription pain medication, only over the counter drugs and a small bag of frozen peas, to manage the pain. Moving was challenging the first week, but several weeks later I started with a physical therapist specializing in women's issues, so I could resume sexual activity.

Since I was post-menopausal, when I had healed from surgery, my doctor prescribed a local estrogen to be inserted directly into the vagina to prevent atrophy. A short time later, however, the vaginal burning returned along with some minor discharge. Initially, I was treated for a yeast infection, but the skin remained inflamed. The new diagnosis was vaginitis. I tried to remain positive, but I couldn't help thinking, "When is it going to end?" I immediately stopped using the vaginal estrogen, in case that was the source of the discharge and inflammation, and started using an ultra-potent steroid cream my doctor prescribed. It seemed like a miracle! After about three months, I managed to get the pain under control; however, if I missed an application, I would be set back for at least a week. My comfort required my diligence.

I wish I could say that at this time my life was perfect and I was like so many other women my doctor treated, but within a few months my libido waned again. My blood tests indicated that my androgens were normal, but my estrogens were so low, they were unrecordable. Although my mother was a breast cancer survivor, my concerns about using estrogen therapy were minimal, especially since my blood values were monitored routinely. I was also reminded to see my gynecologist annually for my check up and mammogram. So I was completely at ease with taking low doses of oral bioidentical estradiol and progesterone. To manage my lack of libido, I was started on a dopamine agonist. Within one week, I was feeling the positive effects of the added medications.

There have been numerous ups and downs throughout this process. There are still times when I don't want to have sex, and times when sex is fun for both Wayne and me. I maintain a positive attitude by not dwelling on the past. But every new day is a new adventure. I wish I could have gotten help when I was much younger, but I intend to have many more years of wedded bliss.

To learn more about how childbirth, menopause, and vulvodynia can affect sexual health and the therapies prescribed for Lil, refer to Part II: The Science.

Sue's Story

Sometimes I felt like I was just a receptacle.

Sue's Story

Sue is a fifty-five-year-old post-menopausal woman who is co-author of this book. Her story is about her transition through menopause. Each of her sexual health issues were resolved almost immediately because her husband is a sexual medicine physician.

One week after meeting Irwin, I announced to my mother, "I met the man I am going to marry." Five years later we married, and three years after that, had the first of our three children. Like every young couple, we were faced with the issues involved in raising a family. It was difficult to find time for the frequent sex we always enjoyed; children walking into the bedroom tended to "destroy the mood." In addition, we both put in a lot of working hours—Irwin in his practice, and me running a household and managing the challenging schedules of three very active children. In spite of everything, we always made time for intimacy because our relationship was important to us.

We had a fulfilling sex life, until I approached my fifties. Then sex stopped being fun. It no longer felt like the reciprocal, loving experience that it had been in the past. Sometimes, I felt like I was just a receptacle. Foreplay had become work, as Irwin's touch no longer aroused me. I began avoiding sex when it was easy to avoid. Occasionally, Irwin would tell me to turn on the radio and light the candles, and then we would have sex, but four out of five times, I wouldn't reach orgasm. My sexual experiences had changed, but I knew that at the age of fifty, fifty percent of men have sexual dysfunction, so I concluded that my husband had a problem.

Even though sexual health was a common topic of conversation in our house, I couldn't bring myself to tell my husband that *he* had a problem, because I didn't want to hurt his feelings. When he first started treating women, we had many conversations about how women function sexually, but we never discussed how sex was changing for *me*. Since I was convinced that this was my husband's issue, it never occurred to me that the physical changes that I was going through, as I approached menopause, might be the reason for my lack of sexual response.

Then one day Irwin brought home the FSFI—the Female Sexual Function Index—the questionnaire that he gives to his female patients. He suggested that I "take it for fun." When he looked at my responses he said, "You have FSD!" It was like the sky opened and everything became clear to me. It wasn't my husband; *I* was the one with the problem! It wasn't *his* fault, so discussing it with him wouldn't make him feel guilty or inadequate. Now, I felt comfortable talking with him about the fact that I had been avoiding sex.

In retrospect, I think that this problem had probably gone on for at least a year. I wasn't interested in having sex because I wasn't enjoying it. Physically, I knew that I was peri-menopausal, because I was having night sweats three or four times a week. Needless to say, I blamed my lack of orgasmic response on my exhaustion. Night sweats were the only menopausal symptom of which I was consciously aware, and as disturbing as they were, I felt fortunate that I wasn't experiencing many of the other horrible symptoms of menopause. I wasn't having mood swings, nothing distressing was happening to me, *so I thought*. It never occurred to me that my sexual problems were a result of the hormonal changes that I was undergoing.

Immediately after seeing the results of the FSFI, Irwin told me I needed to have my blood hormone levels measured. I knew that the results of my blood tests would provide us with a definitive diagnosis and treatment plan. It turned out that my estrogen levels were normal, but my androgen levels were so low that they were all unreadable. I knew that low androgens would cause sexual dysfunction and could create problems, such as low desire, decreased lubrication, diminished orgasm, and even painful intercourse. So I started taking dehydroepiandrosterone every day, and soon the night sweats stopped. It was like a miracle, and you couldn't pay me to get off this medication. After about six weeks on dehydroepiandrosterone, and for the first time in over a year, my sex life returned to normal. I was multi-orgasmic again, and sex was once more an enjoyable experience. Although I didn't always have desire, I was always receptive. I felt good, and I had energy. I didn't know if it was the sleep or the medication, but after six months on dehydroepiandrosterone, I noticed that I had an incredible sense of wellbeing. Even my kids couldn't upset me!

In addition to feeling great and having an improved arousal and orgasmic response from androgen therapy, I realized that something else had changed for me. I distinctly remember preparing dinner one evening and calculating a strategy to keep my husband awake. My plan was to light the candles and turn on music. Then like a bolt of lightning it struck me, "Oh, my God—this is desire." I hadn't experienced that feeling in a while when I used to be interested in having sex for several days before my period. That's the only time that I actually remember having sexual desire since early in our relationship. But there I was in the kitchen, wanting to have sex, planning for it and, most importantly, looking forward to it.

I took advantage of my renewed energy by going to the gym, and became more careful about my diet, choosing fruits and nuts over the ever-present candies and chips. My body was firming up and looking better. I was more confident about how I looked in and out of clothes and more aggressive in the bedroom. I was really enjoying sex in my fifties. I was at a point in my life where I knew what I liked, and I knew what I didn't like. I may have been too shy to say it when I was twenty-five, but now I felt comfortable telling my husband what I wanted sexually. With the kids out of the house, we could even have sex on a Sunday afternoon and not worry. Making love had become fun again.

After being on dehydroepiandrosterone for a year and a half, I couldn't believe it when I started having hot flashes. As I thought about it, I realized that sex had been less satisfying over the last several months. This time I justified the fact that sex hadn't been that great because we had been traveling a lot, and things were crazy. Yet, I was having these hot flashes and the night sweats had returned. My body had deceived me. For several months sex hadn't been good, but it just wasn't in my awareness until the hot flashes and night sweats got my attention. While I had lost interest in sex, I was still receptive, despite the fact that I was having trouble reaching orgasm. Now I was angry—I was angry that my great sex life was gone again.

When I realized that something was wrong, I had my blood hormone levels measured again. My dehydroepiandrosterone was normal, but it wasn't converting properly to the other hormones, so my husband added testosterone to my regimen. Seeing my blood values, I realized that my dysfunction would continue to get worse, and that upset me. As I was aging, my biochemistry was changing, so I needed more medications to get me back to where I was when I was younger. Just three days after starting the testosterone gel, the night sweats stopped, as did the hot flashes. Sexually, everything was good for me again. The testosterone worked quickly, but would this "normal" be only temporary, and would I lose my sexual function once more?

As I suspected, "normal" only lasted for about a year, then sex started to be painful. I was post-menopausal now, and for the first time in my life, intercourse was uncomfortable. Over a ten-day period, each time that we had sex I was feeling more and more discomfort, and it eventually got to the point that sex actually hurt. Even using a significant amount of lubrication didn't help. When I told my husband something was wrong with me because it hurt to have sex, he immediately knew that the pain must have been a result of inadequate estrogens. My blood results confirmed the need for estrogen. So my new treatment regimen included a local estrogen inserted directly into the vagina several times a week.

It is amazing to me how several experiences with painful intercourse impact your muscle response because your muscles have memory. After the local estrogen took effect, we tried to have sex again, and I remember lying there, feeling my muscles clamping shut. I had to say to myself, "Relax your muscles, everything is okay, it's not hurting." Although I was no longer feeling pain, I still needed to tell my muscles to relax. I had to do this several times over the first week after starting the estrogen. This was a really good learning experience for me, because it made me realize why women who have had pain with sex need to go for physical therapy to help them to teach their muscles to relax.

My sexual function continued to be good, and as a part of my care, I had blood tests every six months to measure my hormone levels. When the night sweats returned and my arousal response diminished, I knew that it was time to go in for an additional blood test. My results indicated that my androgens were normal as a result of my medications, but my estrogens were unreadable. The only estrogen that I was using was intravaginal, so my husband prescribed a low dose topical bioidentical estrogen, and a very low dose of oral progesterone, plus a topical estrogen cream for my labial and clitoral area. Once again, I knew that the increase in estrogen was effective because the night sweats disappeared immediately. After one month, I had my bloods drawn again because my husband/sexual medicine physician is always concerned about the use of systemic estrogen. The results of the blood tests indicated that my estrogens were now barely readable. Therefore, my concern about any negative outcomes or increasing my risk of breast cancer was minimal. And I had been getting annual mammograms and Pap smears for years. Although I could probably benefit from more estrogens, I felt more comfortable with a small dose. My estrogen levels were very low, but enough to maintain my sexual function. In addition to all the hormones I used regularly, occasionally just before sex I took half a phosphodiesterase type 5 inhibitor. Assuming I was awake enough to enjoy sexual activity, this medication greatly intensified the lubrication, sensitivity, and orgasms I experienced.

In retrospect, I am able to appreciate all the positive outcomes from this treatment for sexual dysfunction. Bone density tests demonstrated to me the benefits of both weight bearing exercise and hormone therapy, as my results went from below the normal range to normal. From personal experience, I know that the medications improved my energy level and sense of wellbeing. I continue to exercise and eat what I call a modified Mediterranean diet, and I weigh less than I did twenty years ago. My post-menopausal regimen of a daily statin and low dose aspirin help maintain my endothelial health. I am told that if I continue this, my heart, my blood vessels, and my sexual function should remain healthy. The androgen and estrogen hormone therapy eliminated hot flashes and night sweats, and now, two years post-menopause, I realize that it has been an easy transition for me. Presently, I am happy, healthy, and feeling good. Sex is great, and I am once again multi-orgasmic. If we are relaxed and not tired, then sex is like it was in our twenties. I spent my whole life raising my kids, doing all the things that I needed to do, and now, I am on the other side of that. It is our time as a couple to be able to have enjoyment. So my message to the women reading this story is don't settle. A healthy sex life makes everything else in life better.

To learn more about how menopause can affect sexual health and the therapies prescribed for Sue, refer to Part II: The Science.

Comments on Courtney

Courtney didn't realize she had never had an orgasm until, at twenty-eight, she met her second husband, David.

Comments on Courtney

In this story, the authors provide commentary on Courtney's situation. Her lack of knowledge of her sexual function was more common than most people would have believed, despite the plethora of available information about sex.

How can a woman in this day and age not know everything there is to know about sex? You can't pass a magazine rack without seeing stories on sex, and how to make it better. So how could a thirty-two-year-old woman, sexually active since seventeen and in her second marriage, not know about an orgasm?

Courtney didn't realize she had never had an orgasm until, at twenty-eight, she met her second husband, David. During her first marriage, like so many other women, she assumed her sexual experience was "normal," until just before the anniversary of her first date with David, when he brought up the topic of sex. He was older, forty-seven, and more experienced than she, but he had his own sexual problems. It is not uncommon for men to suffer from sexual dysfunction, but they are more apt to seek treatment because there are medications available. David had been going to a sexual medicine physician for five years and was happy with the results. Because Courtney had never experienced an orgasm, he wanted her to see his doctor, but she was embarrassed at the idea. This is a common theme among women. Courtney eventually overcame her shyness about discussing sex, and fear about going to a physician who specialized in sexual medicine, and made an appointment.

It is difficult to talk about a subject as intimate as sex even with your partner, let alone a stranger. When Courtney finally went to the doctor, he was kind and patient and reassuring. He explained about hormones, and how they impact sexual function. In Courtney's case, after the doctor received her blood test results, he prescribed androgens. After about a year and half, he added a dopamine agonist to her regimen, and within four months, she experienced her first orgasm. Now she knew what an orgasm was, and what she had been missing.

Good sex makes for a good marriage. Courtney and her husband became closer. And she now felt more comfortable talking with him about sex. David had felt inadequate because he had been unable to satisfy his young wife sexually. Now, Courtney was easily aroused and had an improved sense of wellbeing. Through their newfound intimacy, their marriage grew stronger, and the couple recently celebrated their first wedding anniversary.

To learn more about the therapies prescribed for Courtney, refer to Part II: The Science.

Part II

The Science

Sexual Medicine Overview

Irwin Goldstein, M.D.

Director, Sexual Medicine
Alvarado Hospital, San Diego, California
Editor-in-Chief, The Journal of Sexual Medicine

Sexual Medicine Overview

Your fundamental sexual health rights entitle you to sexual health care so that you may be free of personal distress or bother from sexual health issues.

According to the European Academy of Sexual Medicine, sexual medicine is the branch of medicine concerned with human sexuality and its disorders. Sexual medicine attempts to improve sexual health through the prevention, diagnosis, treatment, and rehabilitation of conditions or diseases that involve sexual function, sexual and/or partnership experience and behavior, gender identity, and sexual trauma and its consequences. Sexual medicine takes into account the individual and couple dimension, as well as the knowledge and methods of medical, psychological, and social sciences. It recognizes that many of the conditions or disorders may be caused by other medical conditions and/or their treatment.

As discovered by the women in *When Sex Isn't Good*, sexual health problems are unfortunately common. Based on recent studies, it is estimated that, in the United States, more than 10% to 20% of women have problems with sexual desire, arousal, orgasm, and/or pain associated with personal distress or bother. Furthermore, sexual health problems are shared between the genders. A woman whose male partner has an erection problem is very likely to have related reductions in her sexual function and sexual satisfaction. Sexual solutions are also shared. A woman whose partner receives safe and effective treatment for his sexual problem will very likely experience improvement in her sexual function and sexual satisfaction.

It was difficult for the women in *When Sex Isn't Good* to find adequate sexual health care because of the lack of specialists treating women's sexual health issues, be they biologic, psychologic and/or relationship based. Why is this so? The answer is complicated and multi-factorial. Sadly, sexual medicine is not currently a part of the curriculum in most medical schools. Sexual medicine treatment facilities in medical centers are extremely rare. A recurrent and regrettable cycle exists. Practicing healthcare providers received limited information in sexual medicine during their training, leaving them either uncomfortable with the subject or unaware of management options for sexual health problems.

The fact is, though, many individuals and couples, including some healthcare providers themselves, need sexual medicine health care. With the advent of a pill for men, sexual medicine entered the consciousness and conversations of the citizens of the world. Sildenafil was FDA approved as a safe and effective treatment for men with erectile dysfunction in 1998. Since then, it has become "acceptable" for a man to have a sexual health problem, for the sexual health problem to be associated with distress, and for the sexual health problem to be safely and effectively managed by a healthcare provider. The growth of healthcare professionals examining issues in sexual medicine for women is directly related to the release of government-approved, safe and effective treatments for sexual health concerns of men. As more men became aware of help, more women sought help for their unaddressed sexual health concerns.

Efforts should be made by the healthcare professional to resolve the sexual problem with use of the least invasive and most reversible treatment options. If the problem persists, then a step care approach should be utilized engaging therapies that provide benefits, although there are associated risks. As in other aspects of medicine, the sexual medicine healthcare professional and the patient increasingly rely on management principles based on data from well-described, randomized clinical trials, cohort and case-control studies, and meta analyses and/or other systematic review, published in peer review journals that employ principles of evidence-based medicine. The idea is that management principles are not based on personal anecdotal experience.

As evidenced by the many stories in *When Sex Isn't Good*, women with sexual health problems should consider undergoing a diagnostic process which may include a psychologic interview; a history evaluation of potential sexual, medical, and psychosocial concerns; a physical examination, especially of the vestibule; completion of validated questionnaires; and laboratory tests as indicated. Upon conclusion of the initial evaluation, and the development of a presumptive diagnosis, patient (and partner) education and a review of the findings should be performed. Initial treatment efforts should be focused on modifying factors that can be reversed, such as lifestyle changes including diet and exercise, medication changes, sex therapy, physical therapy, and lubricants, vibrators, and dilators as needed.

Should the sexual health problem persist, the next level of intervention involves use of medications for treatment of the sexual health concerns. The EMEA, the European equivalent of the FDA, recently approved the transdermal testosterone patch for the treatment of hypoactive sexual desire disorder in bilaterally oophorectomized and hysterectomized (surgically induced menopause) women receiving concomitant estrogen therapy.

It needs to be emphasized that at the time of writing of *When Sex Isn't Good,* there *does not exist* any FDA-approved pharmacologic treatment for women in the United States with sexual health problems. This means that this critical government agency has not officially established the long-term safety or long-term benefits of any drug treatment for use in women with sexual health problems. Drug treatments prescribed by healthcare professionals, as commonly occurs in *When Sex Isn't Good,* are, in fact, currently used in an "off-label" context. It is thus important for the healthcare provider to inform women patients with sexual health problems of this "off-label" use, and provide them with appropriate and current evidence-based information on risks and benefits of each proposed medication. Armed with this information, each patient will be better able to make an educated decision as to the ultimate use of each "off-label" medication in her personal and unique situation.

As depicted in *When Sex Isn't Good,* what are some of the drug treatments available for the management of women with sexual health concerns associated with evidence-based risks and benefits data in peer review literature? These include: sex steroids such as androgens and estrogens, dopamine agonists, vasodilators, topical potent corticosteroids for treatment of vestibular dermatitis conditions, fungal agents for vestibular and vaginal infections, and pain desensitizers. The judicious use of these agents and others, such as anti-depressants or anti-anxiety agents, by the sexual medicine physician or designated consultants for appropriate biologic-based sexual medicine concerns, can be extremely helpful, as recognized by the women portrayed in *When Sex Isn't Good.*

It is important that drug treatments are not overemphasized. Any pharmacologic agents utilized in sexual health care should be used, as appropriate, in conjunction with continued education and continued efforts at modification of reversible factors. In addition, some women with sexual health problems may require invasive therapies such as surgery. Such intervention should only be considered as a last treatment option when initial strategies alone were not successful in resolving the sexual health concern.

Sexual medicine issues are complex. For example, women may have personal distress from lack of sexual interest, thoughts or fantasies. A marked, disparate sexual interest in a relationship is a common and frustrating interpersonal dilemma. In one individual, the problem could be related primarily to anxiety or depression; in another, it could be principally from partner-related abuse; in another, it could be predominately hormonally-based; and in another, it could be associated with sexual pain, burning, and irritation during sexual activity.

Combinations of causes may exist in any individual. Factors that haven't been mentioned yet, such as pregnancy, drug use, childcare, financial strain, medications, post-surgical complications, cancer treatments, etc., might be the principle issues. In sexual medicine and as described in *When Sex Isn't Good*, the key is that every individual seeking help is unique.

In order to resolve the individual's sexual health problems, mind, body, and relationship issues must be considered. Your sexual medicine physician is dedicated to identifying *all* the interdependent factors involved and to solving the unique situation, as rapidly as possible, using evidence-based safe and effective management strategies, starting at the most reversible and least invasive. Through basic science and clinical research, both biological and psychological, this field will continue to progress. Consequently, healthcare providers will have an opportunity, in the future, to understand more about sexual function and dysfunction and therefore more about therapies to help you.

Symptoms and Risk Factors

Women with sexual health concerns have symptoms that can include:

- Diminished desire, interest, thoughts, and/or fantasies for sexual activity
- No thoughts of sexual activity
- Thoughts of how to avoid sexual activity with partner
- Sexual relationship with a marked discrepancy in sexual interest or desire
- Aversion to being touched, no desire to be touched or no enjoyment from being touched by a partner
- Diminished sexual arousal
- Reduced lubrication and/or too much time required for lubrication
- Difficulty achieving orgasm
- Orgasms that are muffled, weak, not intense, of short duration, and/or of poor quality
- Orgasm induced migraine
- Burning, throbbing, disabling, sharp and/or shooting pain associated with sexual activity
- Genital pain not related to sexual activity
- Unrelenting, unwanted genital arousal with the constant need to relieve it

Women may be at risk for sexual dysfunction if they:

- Have used or use oral, patch or vaginal ring contraceptives
- Have been treated for infertility
- Have been treated for endometriosis
- Have been treated for uterine fibroids, excessive menstrual bleeding or painful menstruation
- Have given birth
- Take anti-depressant, anti-psychotic or anti-anxiety medications
- Take anti-hypertensive medication
- Use recreational/non-prescription drugs
- Are a breast cancer or cervical cancer survivor, especially if treated with chemotherapy and/or anti-hormone therapy
- Are a survivor of other forms of cancer
- Have had a hysterectomy, especially including removal of both ovaries
- Are peri- or post-menopausal
- Have medical problems such as coronary artery disease, diabetes, metabolic syndrome, multiple sclerosis, peripheral neuropathy, spinal cord injury or thyroid disease
- Are in a relationship with an abusive partner
- Have been sexually abused
- Are in a relationship with a partner with erectile dysfunction and/or premature ejaculation
- Are not in a relationship

Effects Of Medical Factors on Sexual Function

Irwin Goldstein, M.D.

Director, Sexual Medicine
Alvarado Hospital, San Diego, California
Editor-in-Chief, The Journal of Sexual Medicine

Anti-Depressants

Psychiatric disorders result in considerable suffering, disability, and healthcare costs. Depressive disorders are associated with feelings of sadness, dejection, and occasional thoughts of suicide. They are also associated with reduced vitality and physical activity, lack of energy, poor ability to concentrate, and inability to sleep. Unfortunately, women are more likely than men to suffer from depression. Studies report that the lifetime prevalence of major depressive disorder is approximately 15%.

Healthcare providers commonly prescribe anti-depressant medications for the safe and effective treatment of depression. Sadly, sexual dysfunction side effects may occur in 15% to 70% of women using anti-depressant medications. Symptoms of anti-depressant-induced sexual dysfunctions include: diminished interest, decreased thoughts and fantasies for sexual activity, diminished sexual arousal and lubrication, and delayed, reduced or absent orgasm. In various publications based on women using anti-depressant therapy, sexual health concerns were commonly reported. For many of these women, sexual function was important. Risk factors for having anti-depressant-induced sexual side effects vary in different studies but commonly include age, less education, obesity, a higher dose of anti-depressants, and a history of cigarette smoking. While some of the anti-depressant drugs are more likely to cause sexual dysfunction, studies showed that the adverse sexual consequences are a "class effect," and that all are at least capable of inducing sexual side effects. The impact of the sexual side effects often makes depressed patients choose to discontinue the important anti-depressant treatment.

The mechanisms whereby the anti-depressants cause sexual side effects are not fully understood, but most researchers in the field believe that the cause is, in part, related to changes in chemicals in the brain. The anti-depressants raise the level of chemical serotonin, a strong inhibitor of sexual activity. There is an associated fall in dopamine, a chemical that is a recognized promoter of sexual interest and orgasm. Some others believe that the anti-depressants also reduce testosterone levels, thereby causing the individual to have drug-induced hormonal sexual problems.

What can you do if you require anti-depressants for depression management and unfortunately get the sexual side effects that cause you personal distress? There are several strategies that you can discuss with your healthcare provider. Your healthcare provider can, for example: reduce the dose of the anti-depressant; take you off the medication for a short period of time; try and substitute with a different anti-depressant; use an anti-depressant that raises the brain chemical dopamine (buproprion); use an anti-depressant that treats the depression via a different mechanism (not by raising serotonin); measure hormones, such as testosterone and estradiol, and consider hormone therapy if the values are low; and consider an antidote such as sildenafil.

References for Anti-depressants:

Althof SE, Leiblum SR, Chevret-Measson M, Hartmann U, Levine SB, McCabe M, Plaut M, Rodrigues O, Wylie K. Psychological and interpersonal dimensions of sexual function and dysfunction. J Sex Med. 2005;2:793–800. Annotation: Medical and psychological therapies for sexual dysfunctions should address bio-psycho-social influences of the patient, the partner, and the couple. No single intervention (i.e., a phosphodiesterase type 5 inhibitor, hormone therapy, processing of childhood victimization, marital therapy, pharmacotherapy for depression, etc.) will be sufficient for most patients or couples experiencing sexual dysfunction.

Andrade L, Caraveo-Anduaga JJ, Berglund P, Bijl RV, De Graaf R, Vollebergh W, Dragomirecka E, Kohn R, Keller M, Kessler RC, Kawakami N, Kilic C, Offord D, Ustun TB, Wittchen HU. The epidemiology of major depressive episodes: results from the International Consortium of Psychiatric Epidemiology (ICPE) Surveys. Int J Methods Psychiatr Res. 2003;12:3–21. Annotation: Face to face studies were carried out in 10 countries, in North America, Latin America, Europe, and Asia, in more than 37,000 subjects. Lifetime prevalence estimates of major depressive episodes varied widely, from 3% in Japan to 16.9% in the United States, with the majority in the range of 8% to 12%. Being female and unmarried were associated risks.

Baldwin DS. Sexual dysfunction associated with antidepressant drugs. Expert Opin Drug Saf. 2004;3:457–70. Annotation: Sexual dysfunction is common in the general population but more common in depressed individuals. There may be some advantages for non-selective serotonin reuptake inhibitor-based anti-depressants, such as bupropion, moclobemide, nefazodone, and reboxetine, over other selective serotonin reuptake inhibitor anti-depressants. Approaches or management of patients with sexual dysfunction associated with anti-depressant treatment include individual and couple psychotherapy, delaying the intake of anti-depressants until after sexual activity, reduction in daily dosage, "drug holidays," use of adjuvant treatments, and switching to a different anti-depressant.

Basson R, Brotto LA, Laan E, Redmond G, Utian WH. Assessment and management of women's sexual dysfunctions: problematic desire and arousal. J Sex Med. 2005;2:291–300. Annotation: Women's sexual response can be re-conceptualized as a circular model of overlapping phases influenced by psychological, societal, and biological factors. Recommendations regarding assessment and management focus on factors reducing arousability and satisfaction, such as a woman's mental health and feelings for her partner, in general, and at the time of sexual activity. Recommendations reflect the poor correlation of subjective arousal and increases in genital vasocongestion.

Clayton AH, Pradko JF, Croft HA, Montano CB, Leadbetter RA, Bolden-Watson C, Bass KI, Donahue RM, Jamerson BD, Metz A. Prevalence of sexual dysfunction among newer antidepressants. J Clin Psychiatry. 2002;63:357–66. Annotation: A total of 4,534 women receiving anti-depressant monotherapy were enrolled. In the overall population, bupropion SR (25%) and nefazodone (28%) were associated with the lowest risk for sexual dysfunction. Selective serotonin reuptake inhibitor anti-depressants, mirtazapine and venlafaxine XR, were associated with higher rates (36% to 43%). In a prospectively defined subpopulation unlikely to have predisposing factors for sexual dysfunction, the prevalence of sexual dysfunction ranged from 7% to 30%, with the odds of having sexual dysfunction 4 to 6 times greater with selective serotonin reuptake inhibitors or venlafaxine XR than with bupropion SR.

Clayton AH. Female sexual dysfunction related to depression and antidepressant medications. Curr Womens Health Rep. 2002;2:182–7. Annotation: Major depression is associated with sexual dysfunction in over 70% of patients. The anti-depressant medications used to treat the illness may exacerbate pre-existing sexual dysfunction or induce sexual dysfunction not present on diagnosis. Strategies to manage sexual dysfunction include switching to anti-depressants with minimal sexual side effects, addition of hormones and/or antidotes, and lowering the dose of medication.

Clayton AH, Zajecka J, Ferguson JM, Filipiak-Reisner JK, Brown MT, Schwartz GE. Lack of sexual dysfunction with the selective noradrenaline reuptake inhibitor reboxetine during treatment for major depressive disorder. Int Clin Psychopharmacol. 2003;18:151–6. Annotation: A total of 450 patients diagnosed with major depressive disorder participated. Reboxetine, a selective noradrenaline reuptake inhibitor, was similar to placebo and superior to fluoxetine, a selective serotonin reuptake inhibitor, in its effect on overall sexual function. There was a greater degree of sexual satisfaction in the reboxetine group compared to fluoxetine. During the study period, female patients able to achieve orgasm increased among those who received reboxetine and placebo but decreased for those who received fluoxetine. These results suggest that reboxetine may be of particular benefit for patients at risk for sexual dysfunction with selective serotonin reuptake inhibitors.

Clayton AH, Warnock JK, Kornstein SG, Pinkerton R, Sheldon-Keller A, McGarvey EL. A placebo-controlled trial of bupropion SR as an antidote for selective serotonin reuptake inhibitor-induced sexual dysfunction. J Clin Psychiatry. 2004;65:62–7. Annotation: A total of 42 patients with selective serotonin reuptake inhibitor-induced sexual dysfunction were randomly assigned to receive either bupropion SR 150 mg twice a day or placebo for 4 weeks in addition to the selective serotonin reuptake inhibitor. Bupropion SR produced an increase in desire to engage in sexual activity and in frequency of engaging in sexual activity, compared with placebo.

Clayton AH, Montejo AL. Major depressive disorder, antidepressants, and sexual dysfunction. J Clin Psychiatry. 2006;67(Suppl 6):33–7. Annotation: Sexual dysfunction is a common problem in patients using anti-depressant medications, especially selective serotonin reuptake inhibitors. Data from a number of studies indicate that non-selective serotonin reuptake inhibitor anti-depressants, such as bupropion, nefazodone, and mirtazapine, alleviate symptoms of sexual dysfunction and are as effective as selective serotonin reuptake inhibitors at controlling depressive symptoms.

Clayton AH, Croft HA, Horrigan JP, Wightman DS, Krishen A, Richard NE, Modell JG. Bupropion extended release compared with escitalopram: effects on sexual functioning and antidepressant efficacy in 2 randomized, double-blind, placebo-controlled studies. J Clin Psychiatry. 2006;67:736–46. Annotation: A study was performed in adults with major depressive disorder and normal sexual functioning. Subjects were randomly assigned bupropion XL, escitalopram or placebo, for up to 8 weeks. The incidence of orgasm dysfunction and the incidence of worsened sexual functioning at the end of the treatment period were significantly lower with bupropion XL than with escitalopram, not different between bupropion XL and placebo, and significantly higher with escitalopram than with placebo.

Delgado PL, Brannan SK, Mallinckrodt CH, Tran PV, McNamara RK, Wang F, Watkin JG, Detke MJ. Sexual functioning assessed in 4 double-blind placebo- and paroxetine-controlled trials of duloxetine for major depressive disorder. J Clin Psychiatry. 2005;66:686–92. Annotation: A total of 1,466 patients with major depressive disorder were assigned to receive placebo, duloxetine or paroxetine. In female patients, sexual dysfunction was significantly less in the non-selective serotonin reuptake inhibitor-based duloxetine treatment group, compared with the selective serotonin reuptake inhibitor paroxetine treatment group. Both rates were significantly higher than placebo.

Foley KF, DeSanty KP, Kast RE. Bupropion: pharmacology and therapeutic applications. Expert Rev Neurother. 2006;6:1249–65. Annotation: Bupropion is a safe and effective anti-depressant, suitable for first-line use in major depression and seasonal affective disorder. Common side effects are nervousness and insomnia, with a predominant concern for seizures in those with a history of seizures. Bupropion, a dopamine agonist, is effective in helping people quit tobacco smoking. Sexual dysfunction with bupropion use is probably the least of any anti-depressant.

Hasin DS, Goodwin RD, Stinson FS, Grant BF. Epidemiology of major depressive disorder: results from the National Epidemiologic Survey on Alcoholism and Related Conditions. Arch Gen Psychiatry. 2005;62:1097–106. Annotation: Face to face studies of more than 43,000 adults aged 18 years and older, residing in the United States, revealed a prevalence of lifetime major depressive disorder of 13%. Being female, middle-aged, widowed, separated or divorced, and low income increased risk. Women were also significantly more likely to receive treatment than men.

Heo M, Pietrobelli A, Fontaine KR, Sirey JA, Faith MS. Depressive mood and obesity in US adults: comparison and moderation by sex, age, and race. Int J Obes (Lond). 2006;30:513–9. Annotation: A total of 44,800 respondents to a national survey were studied. The prevalence of depressive mood was 14%. Young, overweight, and obese women were significantly more likely to have experienced depressive mood than non-overweight/non-obese women. Young, obese women were also significantly more likely to have a sustained depressive mood than non-overweight/non-obese women.

Kennedy SH, Eisfeld BS, Dickens SE, Bacchiochi JR, Bagby RM. Antidepressant-induced sexual dysfunction during treatment with moclobemide, paroxetine, sertraline, and venlafaxine. J Clin Psychiatry. 2000;61:276-81. Annotation: Disturbances in sexual function were assessed in 107 patients who met criteria for major depressive disorder and received treatment with moclobemide, paroxetine, sertraline or venlafaxine. The reported impairment in drive/desire items for women ranged from 26% to 32%. Rates of sexual dysfunction in women were generally higher with sertraline and paroxetine, but only significantly so in comparison with moclobemide on some measures.

Kennedy SH, Fulton KA, Bagby RM, Greene AL, Cohen NL, Rafi-Tari S. Sexual function during bupropion or paroxetine treatment of major depressive disorder. Can J Psychiatry. 2006;51:234–42. Annotation: A total of 141 patients (68 women) with major depressive episodes were randomly assigned to receive bupropion SR or paroxetine, under double-blind trial conditions. There was a significant inverse relation between depression and sexual function in women. A significant difference in anti-depressant-related sexual dysfunction was detected in men, but not women, during treatment with bupropion SR or paroxetine.

Kessler RC, Berglund P, Demler O, Jin R, Koretz D, Merikangas KR, Rush AJ, Walters EE, Wang PS. The epidemiology of major depressive disorder: results from the National Comorbidity Survey Replication (NCS-R). JAMA. 2003;289:3095–105. Annotation: A face-to-face survey was conducted in over 9,000 residents, ages 18 years or older. The prevalence of major depressive disorder for lifetime was 16%. Major depressive disorder is common, widely distributed in the population, and usually associated with substantial symptom severity and role impairment.

Nurnberg HG, Hensley PL. Selective phosphodiesterase type-5 inhibitor treatment of serotonergic reuptake inhibitor antidepressant-associated sexual dysfunction: a review of diagnosis, treatment, and relevance. CNS Spectr. 2003;8:194–202. Annotation: Sexual dysfunction secondary to selective serotonin reuptake inhibitor use is a major cause of premature treatment discontinuation. Sexual function should be evaluated prior to the anti-depressant disturbances related to the depression and prior to changes associated with anti-depressant treatment. Inquiry should also be made for concurrent medical conditions, somatic treatments, lifestyle risk factors, and response to anti-depressants.

Shen WW, Urosevich Z, Clayton DO. Sildenafil in the treatment of female sexual dysfunction induced by selective serotonin reuptake inhibitors. J Reprod Med. 1999;44:535–42. Annotation: Literature reviews of published articles were done. Sildenafil may be beneficial in reversing female sexual dysfunction induced by selective serotonin reuptake inhibitors.

Williams VS, Baldwin DS, Hogue SL, Fehnel SE, Hollis KA, Edin HM. Estimating the prevalence and impact of antidepressant-induced sexual dysfunction in 2 European countries: a cross-sectional patient survey. J Clin Psychiatry. 2006;67:204–10. Annotation: A survey of 502 adults in France and the United Kingdom was performed. It revealed that 27% of the French sample and 39% of the UK sample were classified as having anti-depressant-induced sexual dysfunction. Patients with anti-depressant-induced sexual dysfunction reported that changes in sexual functioning negatively affected their self-esteem, mood, and relationships with sexual partners.

Cancer Treatment

Sexual activity is probably the last thing on your mind when you hear the word "cancer." No matter what type of cancer you have, it can negatively affect your emotions. The many possible treatments, such as radiation, surgery, chemotherapy, and hormone ablation therapies, carry the risk of causing physical changes to your body that may result in sexual dysfunction.

Women being treated for breast or gynecologic cancers are most likely to experience side effects consistent with reduced sexual interest, reduced arousal, reduced lubrication, absent or muted orgasm, and increased sexual pain. The treatment received and type and stage of cancer will impact the extent of sexual side effects. Treatments can affect self-esteem and self-worth, impacting your attitude toward sexual activity and intimacy with your partner. Once you complete treatment, you may wish to resume sexual activity. For some women, this may be important in order to help feel intimate and sexual again.

A total of 8% to 10% of women will be diagnosed with breast cancer, a quarter of whom will be pre-menopausal. Psychological and physical factors of the breast cancer may adversely affect body image and sexual relationship. Body image may be influenced by stage of cancer, type of breast surgery, chemotherapy, lymphedema, hair loss, surgical menopause, and age at diagnosis. After breast surgery, many women report impaired or unpleasant physical sensations in their breasts. Almost half of women with partial mastectomy and over 80% of those with breast reconstruction report decreased pleasure from breast caressing. Loss of breast sensitivity may contribute to further loss of sexual interest.

Chemotherapy is often associated with loss of interest in sexual activity. The nausea, hair loss, and weight loss or gain can make a woman feel unattractive. Chemotherapy can cause early onset menopause and a sudden loss of ovarian estrogen production. Menopausal symptoms, such as vaginal atrophy and vaginal dryness, can cause pain during vaginal penetration. Depending on cancer type, estrogen therapy, either local or systemic, may be prescribed to help reduce sexual side effects of chemotherapy-induced menopause. A plan of judicious use of local estrogen therapy with repeated hormone blood testing may be discussed with healthcare providers.

Hormone ablation therapy may be utilized if the breast cancer is hormone-sensitive. One of the drugs commonly used is tamoxifen, usually taken for 5 years. Tamoxifen, itself, may increase the incidence of sexual dysfunction. Limited studies indicate that tamoxifen treatment is associated with decreased sexual interest and increased vaginal dryness. In a study designed to specifically assess the effects of tamoxifen on sexual function in women, more than half of sexually active women with breast cancer on tamoxifen experienced sexual pain during intercourse unrelated to previous chemotherapy. Breast cancer patients treated with tamoxifen as adjuvant therapy may exhibit symptoms of estrogen deprivation, including sexual dysfunction related to alterations in vaginal tissue structure and function. In a recent animal study, tamoxifen use was associated with decreased vaginal blood flow following sexual stimulation and an inability of the vaginal lining cells to release the mucin protein that helps quality of vaginal lubrication.

Pre-existing sexual disorders may be made worse by the menopausal loss of estrogens. Another biologic cause of arousal difficulties is pelvic floor spasm as a result of vaginal dryness and dyspareunia. Learning pelvic floor relaxation and encouraging self-massage with medicated oil may effectively relieve dyspareunia and arousal disorders, secondary to diminished blood levels of estrogen.

Women with breast cancer are unable to receive systemic estrogen treatment because of the risk of breast cancer recurrence. Topical vaginal estrogen treatments may be considered as an option, however you and your oncologist should make this decision together, after you have been informed of the risks and benefits. Women with good sexual interest but genital arousal disorders may have some clinical improvement with oral phosphodiesterase type 5 inhibitors (e.g., sildenafil), not contraindicated in breast cancer patients, for increased arousal. In addition, dopamine agonists such as buproprion are not contraindicated in breast cancer patients and may be prescribed to improve desire.

All women are born with the breast cancer genes 1 and 2 (BRCA). When functioning normally, these genes do not pose any risk to a woman's health. However, some women may be born with or experience mutations of the BRCA genes in their lifetime. Women who have BRCA mutations are at increased risk for developing breast and ovarian cancers, compared with women who do not have these mutations. A 30-year-old woman with a BRCA mutation has a 1 in 3 chance of developing breast cancer during her lifetime, compared with a 1 in 8 chance for a woman without these genetic mutations. Over a lifetime, women with BRCA mutations have a 50% to 85% chance of developing ovarian cancer. Women who test positive for BRCA mutations may consider breast cancer prevention with the drug tamoxifen or undergo prophylactic removal of the breasts. To lower the chances of ovarian cancer, women who test positive for BRCA mutations may consider taking birth control pills for at least 5 years or undergo ovarian removal. Testing positive for BRCA mutations does not guarantee that a woman will develop breast cancer or ovarian cancer, however prophylactic therapies can affect sexual function.

There are many other ways in which cancer treatments cause sexual side effects. Radiation therapy to cancers in the pelvic region, such as bladder, cervical, colon, rectal, and ovarian cancer, may cause several sexual side effects. The strength of radiation treatments may cause them to damage the ovaries. Surgery may be considered to relocate the ovaries to another part of the body. This might spare them from the damage of radiation and early menopause, and potentially preserve fertility. Damaged ovaries that do not produce estrogen may leave women in radiation-associated menopause with the classic symptoms of vaginal dryness, night sweats, and hot flashes. Radiation to the pelvis may also cause changes in the vagina and irritate nearby vaginal tissue, causing the lining of the vagina to become inflamed and tender. Penetration during sex may be uncomfortable during such cancer treatment. In some cancers, reduced size of the vagina may be an issue post-treatment. As the lining of the vagina heals, thickening and scarring may cause it to tighten and resist stretching during penetration. Use of a vaginal dilator may help prevent scar tissue from forming in the vagina after radiation.

Surgery for cancer of the various genital or pelvic organs may also cause sexual side effects. Radical hysterectomy, the removal of the uterus and related ligaments, as well as the cervix and part of the vagina, is performed in some women with cervical or uterine cancers. A shortened vagina may result postoperatively. Women may also have their ovaries removed during this surgery, in which case surgical menopause and subsequent vaginal atrophy will result.

Radical cystectomy, the removal of the bladder, uterus, ovaries, fallopian tubes, cervix, front wall of the vagina, and urethra may be considered in women with bladder cancer. A reconstructed vagina may be shorter or narrower postoperatively. Sex may be painful because of these changes to the vagina and because of the surgical menopause that induces vaginal atrophy.

Abdominoperineal resection, the removal of the lower colon and rectum, may be performed for colon or rectal cancer. Without the rectum, a woman may experience pain in her vagina during penetration. Some women who have an abdominoperineal resection also have their ovaries removed, in which case surgical menopause and vaginal atrophy will result. Vulvectomy, removal of the entire vulva, including the labia majora and labia minora as well as the clitoris, is performed for cancer of the vulva. Removing the vulva and clitoris will result in a less sensitive vestibule leading to muted orgasm during sexual activity.

The diagnosis and treatments provided to woman with cancer, especially breast cancer, may have a strong effect on a woman's sexual identity, sexual function, and sexual relationship. Cancer survivors and their partners may need sexual counseling and carefully thought out biologic treatments that do not encourage cancer growth but can improve the quality of intimacy, body image, and sexual relationship.

References for Cancer Treatment:

Amsterdam A, Krychman ML. Sexual dysfunction in patients with gynecologic neoplasms: a retrospective pilot study. J Sex Med. 2006;3:646–9. Annotation: A total of 259 female cancer patients attending a survivorship program participated. Symptomatic treatment recommendations included hormone therapy alternatives, psychosexual counseling, local vaginal estrogen suppositories, and vaginal dilators. The most frequent presenting complaints encountered were dyspareunia (72%), atrophic vaginitis (65%), hypoactive desire (43%), and orgasmic dysfunction (17%). At a median of 6 months, 60 patients (63%) received follow-up, and of them, 42 (70%) self-reported improvement in their symptoms.

Avis NE, Crawford S, Manuel J. Quality of life among younger women with breast cancer. J Clin Oncol. 2005;23:3322–30. Annotation: A total of 202 women diagnosed with breast cancer at age 50 or younger were studied. Unhappiness with appearance was reported by more than 70% of women. Pain with sexual intercourse significantly increased with age. Quality of life was significantly lower than compared to a non-patient sample of women. Relationship, sexual and body image problems after diagnosis, vaginal dryness, and feeling unprepared for the impact of breast cancer were associated with quality of life issues.

Baber R, Hickey M, Kwik M. Therapy for menopausal symptoms during and after treatment for breast cancer: safety considerations. Drug Saf. 2005;28:1085–100. Annotation: Breast cancer is the most common newly diagnosed cancer in women. Lifetime risk in the United States is 1 in 8, in the United Kingdom, 1 in 9, and in Australia, 1 in 11 women, of whom approximately 27% will be pre-menopausal at the time of their diagnosis. Many of these women will experience a sudden menopause as a result of chemotherapy, endocrine therapy or surgical interventions. Non-hormonal treatments may also be considered, including clonidine, gabapentin, and some anti-depressants. Various selective serotonin reuptake inhibitors may be considered. The largest randomized trial examining the relationship between post-menopausal hormone therapy and breast cancer recurrence was recently halted because of a reported increase in the risk of recurrence among users of hormone therapy.

Burwell SR, Case LD, Kaelin C, Avis NE. Sexual problems in younger women after breast cancer surgery. J Clin Oncol. 2006;24:2815–21. Annotation: In 209 women sexually active at baseline (78.6% of total sample), sexual problems were significantly greater immediately post-surgery and at 1 year post-surgery, compared to before breast cancer diagnosis. Pre-diagnoses of vaginal dryness and lower perceived sexual attractiveness were consistently related to greater overall sexual problems. Women who became menopausal as a result of chemotherapy continued to have sexual problems.

Butler-Manuel SA, Buttery LD, A'Hern RP, Polak JM, Barton DP. Pelvic nerve plexus trauma at radical hysterectomy and simple hysterectomy: the nerve content of the uterine supporting ligaments. Cancer. 2000;89:834–41. Annotation: A total of 31 women undergoing hysterectomy also underwent intraoperative cross-sectional biopsies to determine the nerve content of the removed utero-sacral ligaments. Autonomic nerves and ganglia were identified in the uterine supporting ligament specimen of women undergoing hysterectomy. These data provide evidence for nerve damage associated with hysterectomy surgery.

Butler-Manuel SA, Buttery LD, A'Hern RP, Polak JM, Barton DP. Pelvic nerve plexus trauma at radical and simple hysterectomy: a quantitative study of nerve types in the uterine supporting ligaments. J Soc Gynecol Investig. 2002;9:47–56. Annotation: Cross-sectional biopsies were collected from the uterine insertion of these ligaments in 11 women who had a simple hysterectomy for benign disease. Autonomic nerves are transected in the lateral division of the uterine supporting ligaments during a simple hysterectomy. Sympathetic, parasympathetic, sensory, and sensory-motor nerve types are present within uterine supporting ligaments. The uterine supporting ligaments are a major pathway for autonomic nerves to the pelvic organs.

Ganz PA, Rowland JH, Meyerowitz BE, Desmond KA. Impact of different adjuvant therapy strategies on quality of life in breast cancer survivors. Recent Results Cancer Res. 1998;152:396–411. Annotation: A total of 1,098 women, diagnosed between 1 and 5 years before with early stage breast cancer, were studied. Sexual functioning scores did differ with patients receiving chemotherapy, either alone or with tamoxifen, experiencing more problems. Hot flashes, night sweats, and vaginal discharge were reported more often in breast cancer survivors on tamoxifen. Vaginal dryness and pain with intercourse also differed significantly by adjuvant treatment, occurring more often in survivors treated with chemotherapy. Compared to survivors with no adjuvant therapy, those who received chemotherapy have significantly more sexual problems.

Ganz PA, Greendale GA, Petersen L, Kahn B, Bower JE. Breast cancer in younger women: reproductive and late health effects of treatment. J Clin Oncol. 2003;21:4184–93. Annotation: A total of 577 women were surveyed approximately 6 years after diagnosis. Amenorrhea occurred frequently as a result of treatment, and treatment-associated menopause was associated with poorer health perceptions. The youngest women experienced poorer mental health and less vitality. Better outcomes were observed in married or partnered women, and women with better emotional and physical functioning. Factors that contribute to poorer quality of life include experiencing a menopausal transition as part of therapy and feeling more vulnerable after cancer.

Hendren SK, O'Connor BI, Liu M, Asano T, Cohen Z, Swallow CJ, Macrae HM, Gryfe R, McLeod RS. Prevalence of male and female sexual dysfunction is high following surgery for rectal cancer. Ann Surg. 2005;242:212–23. Annotation: A total of 81 women treated for rectal cancer participated. Current sexual activity was significantly less post-operatively, 32%, versus 61% pre-operatively. Current sexual activity was associated with present age, surgical procedure, and pre-operative sexual activity. "Surgery made sexual life worse" was reported by 29% of women, and associated with surgical procedure and radiation therapy. Sexual problems were decreased sexual interest 41%, arousal 29%, lubrication 56%, orgasm 35%, and dyspareunia 46%. Women reported a negative body image. Patients seldom remembered discussing sexual risks pre-operatively or being treated for dysfunction post-operatively.

Hickey M, Saunders CM, Stuckey BG. Management of menopausal symptoms in patients with breast cancer: an evidence-based approach. Lancet Oncol. 2005;6:687–95. Annotation: Increasing numbers of women have menopausal symptoms after treatment for breast cancer secondary to the cancer treatments, such as oophorectomy, chemotherapy-induced ovarian failure, and anti-estrogens, or after discontinuation of hormone therapy. These menopausal symptoms can have an effect on sexual function and self-esteem. Selective inhibitors of serotonin and norepinephrine reuptake seem to offer reasonable symptom palliation, but the long-term effectiveness and safety of these preparations is not known.

Jensen PT, Groenvold M, Klee MC, Thranov I, Petersen MA, Machin D. Longitudinal study of sexual function and vaginal changes after radiotherapy for cervical cancer. Int J Radiat Oncol Biol Phys. 2003;56:937–49. Annotation: A total of 118 patients referred for radiation therapy were studied. Sexual dysfunction and adverse vaginal changes were reported throughout the 2 years after radiation therapy, with small changes over time: approximately 85% had low or no sexual interest, 35% had moderate to severe lack of lubrication, 55% had mild to severe dyspareunia, and 30% were dissatisfied with their sexual life. A reduced vaginal dimension was reported by 50% of the patients.

Krychman ML. Sexual rehabilitation medicine in a female oncology setting. Gynecol Oncol. 2006;101:380–4. Annotation: Comprehensive oncological care now includes survivorship medicine to help male and female cancer patients live active, fulfilled lives. Specialized sexual health programs address cancer patients' sexual needs based on patient education and support, medical and scientific research, and medical education and training for health care professionals and providers.

Sheppard C, Whiteley R. Psychosexual problems after gynaecological cancer. J Br Menopause Soc. 2006;12:24–7. Annotation: Sexual difficulties may persist long after the cancer has successfully been treated. Gynecological cancers affect a woman's body image and her fear of dying. A couple's sexual relationship often changes focus from partners/lovers to "patient and career."

Speer JJ, Hillenberg B, Sugrue DP, Blacker C, Kresge CL, Decker VB, Zakalik D, Decker DA. Study of sexual functioning determinants in breast cancer survivors. Breast J. 2005;11:440–7. Annotation: A total of 55 female breast cancer survivors participated. Sexual functioning was significantly poorer in breast cancer survivors than published normal controls. Relationship distress level affected arousal, orgasm, lubrication, satisfaction, and sexual pain. Depression was a determinant of low sexual desire. Breast cancer survivors on anti-depressants had higher levels of arousal dysfunction and orgasm dysfunction. Women who were older had significantly more concerns about vaginal lubrication and pain.

Thranov I, Klee M. Sexuality among gynecologic cancer patients—a cross-sectional study. Gynecol Oncol. 1994;52:14–9. Annotation: All 146 patients had gynecologic cancer treated with chemotherapy or radiation therapy. Little or no desire for sexual relations was found among 74% of the patients and 42% of their partners. Among the sexually active patients, 40% experienced dyspareunia.

Childbirth

One of the poorly recognized risk factors for long-term female sexual dysfunction is childbirth. It is not uncommon in a clinic to hear a woman complain that her sex life never returned to normal after giving birth. The expectation of most mothers is that there will be some changes in sexual function in the immediate post-partum period, but they anticipate an eventual return to normalcy. This may not be the case.

Is childbirth a genuine risk factor for long-term sexual dysfunction? Unfortunately, there are few investigations of this association. These few studies do, however, reveal that long-term sexual dysfunction does develop as a result of childbirth. In one study, six months after childbirth, sexual responsiveness and sexual desire remained reduced in approximately 1 in 4 of the mothers. In another study, at 6 months postpartum, 22% reported painful intercourse. At 13 months postpartum, 1 in 5 women were still having sexual dysfunction. In another study, at 6 months postpartum, approximately 40% of women did not reach pre-pregnancy levels of sexual function. In yet another study, at 6 months postpartum, approximately 1 of 5 women reported dyspareunia, 4 of 10 reported no orgasm, and 1 in 5 reported worsened orgasmic function. After 6 months postpartum, a total of 26% of women complained of loss of sexual desire, 13%, lack of vaginal lubrication, 21%, painful penetration, and 15%, difficulty achieving orgasm.

Risk factors for sexual dysfunction after childbirth include depression, change in partner relationship, fatigue, and 4th degree vaginal tears. Endocrine changes during pregnancy may result in sexual dysfunction. The elevated hormonal changes of pregnancy, such as estradiol values over 1000 pg/ml for 8 of the 9 months, may act to permanently alter the activity of certain critical enzymes in the androgen synthetic pathway necessary for sexual health.

In the long run, the sexual relationship of at least 1/3 of all couples suffers a change for the worse as a result of childbirth. While there is not yet sufficient scientific evidence, these changes appear to be permanent. Sexual medicine specialists can often provide help to women who experience distress as a result of the sexual dysfunction.

References for Childbirth:

Barrett G, Pendry E, Peacock J, Victor C, Thakar R, Manyonda I. Women's sexual health after childbirth. BJOG. 2000;107:186–95. Annotation: A total of 484 primiparous women (having given birth only once) who gave birth in a 6-month period participated. A total of 89% had resumed sexual activity within 6 months of the birth. Sexual morbidity increased significantly after the birth: in the first 3 months after delivery, 83% of women experienced sexual problems, declining to 64% at 6 months. Dyspareunia in the first 3 months after delivery was significantly associated with vaginal deliveries. Only 15% of women who had a post-natal sexual problem reported discussing it with a health professional.

Barrett G, Peacock J, Victor CR, Manyonda I. Cesarean section and postnatal sexual health. Birth. 2005;32:306–11. Annotation: A study was conducted in 796 primiparous women. Any protective effect of cesarean section on sexual function was limited to the early post-natal period, primarily to dyspareunia-related symptoms. At 6 months, the differences in dyspareunia-related symptoms, sexual response-related symptoms, and post-coital problems were much reduced, and none reached statistical significance.

Connolly A, Thorp J, Pahel L. Effects of pregnancy and childbirth on postpartum sexual function: a longitudinal prospective study. Int Urogynecol J Pelvic Floor Dysfunct. 2005;16:263–7. Annotation: A total of 150 women were enrolled who were at 30–40 weeks gestation. At 24 weeks postpartum, 90% of the women had resumed intercourse, 17% of women reported dyspareunia, 39% reported no orgasm, and 17% reported worsened orgasmic function.

Hicks TL, Goodall SF, Quattrone EM, Lydon-Rochelle MT. Postpartum sexual functioning and method of delivery: summary of the evidence. J Midwifery Womens Health. 2004;49:430–6. Annotation: A literature review was performed on selected postpartum sexual function outcomes. The studies all showed increased risks of delay in resumption of intercourse, dyspareunia, sexual problems, or perineal pain, associated with assisted vaginal delivery. Some studies showed less dyspareunia for women with cesarean delivery. An association between assisted vaginal delivery and some degree of sexual dysfunction is reported.

Oboro VO, Tabowei TO. Sexual function after childbirth in Nigerian women. Int J Gynaecol Obstet. 2002;78:249–50. Annotation: After 6 months postpartum, there were new sexual problems reported. Women complained of loss of sexual desire (26%), lack of vaginal lubrication (13%), painful penetration (21%), and difficulty achieving orgasm (15%).

Ryding EL. Sexuality during and after pregnancy. Acta Obstet Gynecol Scand. 1984;63:679–82. Annotation: The effects of pregnancy and childbirth on sexuality were studied in 50 women. Dyspareunia was more common in first time birth mothers. Coital frequency and orgasmic capacity decreased during pregnancy. Three months after childbirth, 20% of the women had little desire for and a further 21% had a complete loss of, desire for or aversion to sexual activity.

van Brummen HJ, Bruinse HW, van de Pol G, Heintz AP, van der Vaart CH. Which factors determine the sexual function 1 year after childbirth? BJOG. 2006;113:914–8. Annotation: A total of 377 nulliparous women (never having given birth) were studied. The main predictive factor for no sexual intercourse 1 year postpartum was no sexual intercourse at 12 weeks of gestation. Women were 5 times less likely to be sexually active after a 3rd/4th degree anal sphincter tear as compared with women with an intact perineum. Dissatisfaction with the sexual relationship 1 year after childbirth was associated with not being sexually active at 12 weeks of gestation and with an older maternal age at delivery.

Diabetes

Sexual health problems, such as decreased interest, slowness to arouse, decreased vaginal lubrication, orgasmic dysfunction, and sexual pain, are reported more often in women with diabetes mellitus than in women without diabetes. For women with diabetes mellitus, researchers have found that psychologic factors, as well as biologic factors such as diabetes-associated damage to nerves and blood vessels, have been implicated as the causes of the sexual health problems.

Several studies have been published on the sexual health concerns of women with diabetes mellitus, although it is obvious that more research is needed. Enzlin and colleagues compared data concerning the sexual health problems of three groups of women: type 1 diabetes mellitus without diabetic complications; type 1 diabetes mellitus with diabetic complications; and an age-matched healthy control group of women without diabetes mellitus. Compared to the healthy women without diabetes mellitus, those women with diabetes had significantly more (approaching twice as many) sexual health problems, significantly higher occurrence of decreased lubrication, and significantly more depressive symptoms. Among the women with diabetes mellitus, a significant association was found between the number of diabetic-related complications and the number of sexual health complaints; women with more diabetic-related complications also reported more sexual health problems.

Erol and colleagues examined the sexual health concerns of women with type 2 diabetes mellitus. Compared to age-matched healthy controls without diabetes mellitus, women with diabetes had significantly lower sexual function scores on a validated questionnaire. The most common sexual health problems in the women with diabetes were reduced libido (almost 4 of 5), diminished clitoral sensation (almost 2 of 3), and increased vaginal dryness and discomfort (almost 2 of 5).

Salonia and colleagues examined women with diabetes mellitus and compared them to a healthy age-matched control group without diabetes mellitus. Compared to healthy women, those with diabetes mellitus had significantly lower sexual function scores in the areas of sexual desire, lubrication, and sexual orgasm and, in addition, had significantly higher sexual pain. Women with diabetes and depression had significantly less arousal, orgasm, and satisfaction compared to those diabetic women without depression. Older diabetic women had less sexual interest and less lubrication than younger diabetic women. Consistent with age being an important factor, Schiel and colleagues reported that the overall prevalence of sexual health problems was twice as common in women with type 2 diabetes mellitus (who are much older) compared to women with type 1 diabetes mellitus (who are younger).

Recent animal studies have shown that diabetes can be associated with abnormalities in structure and function of genital tissues, in particular with nerve and blood vessel damage.

If you are a woman with diabetes mellitus and sexual health problems that are causing personal distress, consultation with a sexual medicine physician is suggested. Diabetes is associated with obvious biologic reasons for sexual dysfunction. Some potential pharmacologic therapies include sex steroids, vasodilators, and dopamine agonists.

References for Diabetes:

Bultrini A, Carosa E, Colpi EM, Poccia G, Iannarelli R, Lembo D, Lenzi A, Jannini EA. Possible correlation between type 1 diabetes mellitus and female sexual dysfunction: case report and literature review. J Sex Med. 2004;1:337–40. Annotation: A 29-year-old white woman observed a sexual arousal disorder of sudden onset, complicated by loss of orgasm and sexual desire, in the absence of any marital, relational, psychological or gynecological cause. One month later, she was diagnosed with severe type 1 diabetes. With the correction of diabetes and without other treatment of the sexual dysfunction, she experienced a full recovery from her sexual complaints. Female sexual dysfunction may be an early symptom of diabetes mellitus, and good glycemic control is fundamental to restore sexual activity in diabetic women.

Caruso S, Rugolo S, Agnello C, Intelisano G, Di Mari L, Cianci A. Sildenafil improves sexual functioning in premenopausal women with type 1 diabetes who are affected by sexual arousal disorder: a double-blind, crossover, placebo-controlled pilot study. Fertil Steril. 2006;85:1496–501. Annotation: Thirty-two type 1 pre-menopausal diabetic women affected by sexual arousal disorder participated. Plasma concentrations of free testosterone were normal. Sildenafil improved arousal, orgasm, sexual enjoyment, and dyspareunia in women affected by type 1 diabetes.

Caruso S, Rugolo S, Mirabella D, Intelisano G, Di Mari L, Cianci A. Changes in clitoral blood flow in premenopausal women affected by type 1 diabetes after single 100-mg administration of sildenafil. Urology. 2006;68:161–5. Annotation: A total of 30 pre-menopausal women with type 1 diabetes treated with insulin therapy and 39 healthy pre-menopausal women participated. Each diabetic woman received a single oral dose of 100 mg sildenafil. Color Doppler ultrasonography was used to measure clitoral blood flow. The baseline clitoral blood flow of the diabetic women was lower, compared with that of the control group. One hour after sildenafil, the clitoral blood flow was significantly greater, compared with baseline.

Doruk H, Akbay E, Cayan S, Akbay E, Bozlu M, Acar D. Effect of diabetes mellitus on female sexual function and risk factors. Arch Androl. 2005;51:1–6. Annotation: The study consisted of 127 married women: 21 with type 1 diabetes, 50 with type 2 diabetes, and 56 healthy controls. The prevalence of sexual dysfunction was 71% in the type 1 diabetic group, 42% in the type 2 diabetic group, and 37% in the control subjects. The scores for sexual desire, arousal, and lubrication were significantly lower in the type 1 diabetes group than in the control subjects.

Enzlin P, Mathieu C, Van den Bruel A, Bosteels J, Vanderschueren D, Demyttenaere K. Sexual dysfunction in women with type 1 diabetes: a controlled study. Diabetes Care. 2002;25:672–7. Annotation: In this study of 120 women with diabetes and 180 age-matched healthy controls, significantly more diabetic woman than control subjects reported decreased lubrication. Diabetic women with sexual dysfunction mentioned lower overall quality of marital relationship and more depressive symptoms than diabetic women without sexual problems.

Enzlin P, Mathieu C, Van Den Bruel A, Vanderschueren D, Demyttenaere K. Prevalence and predictors of sexual dysfunction in patients with type 1 diabetes. Diabetes Care. 2003;26:409–14. Annotation: A total of 240 adult type 1 diabetic patients completed questionnaires. Sexual dysfunction was reported by 27% of women. In women, sexual dysfunction was not related to age, BMI, duration of diabetes or diabetic complications. In women, sexual dysfunction was related to depression and quality of the partner relationship.

Giraldi A, Persson K, Werkstrom V, Alm P, Wagner G, Andersson KE. Effects of diabetes on neurotransmission in rat vaginal smooth muscle. Int J Impot Res. 2001;13:58–66. Annotation: Female rats were divided into two groups: non-diabetic controls and diabetics. Diabetes was shown to interfere with adrenergic, cholinergic, and non-adrenergic non-cholinergic neurotransmitter mechanisms in the smooth muscle of the rat vagina.

Kim NN, Stankovic M, Cushman TT, Goldstein I, Munarriz R, Traish AM. Streptozotocin-induced diabetes in the rat is associated with changes in vaginal hemodynamics, morphology and biochemical markers. BMC Physiol. 2006;6:4. Annotation: Control and diabetic female rats were studied. Diabetic rats had decreased mean body weight and lower levels of plasma estradiol, compared to age-matched controls. The vaginal blood flow response to pelvic nerve stimulation was significantly reduced in diabetic rats. Histological examination of vaginal tissue from diabetic animals showed reduced epithelial thickness and atrophy of the muscularis layer. Diabetes may lead to multiple disruptions in sex steroid hormone synthesis, metabolism, and action. These pathological events may cause changes in both tissue structure and key enzymes that regulate cell growth and smooth muscle contractility, ultimately affecting the genital response during sexual arousal.

Lewis RW, Fugl-Meyer KS, Bosch R, Fugl-Meyer AR, Laumann EO, Lizza E, Martin-Morales A. Epidemiology/risk factors of sexual dysfunction. J Sex Med. 2004;1:35–9. Annotation: The prevalence of sexual dysfunction increases as women age; about 40% to 45% of adult women have at least one manifest sexual dysfunction. Common risk factor categories associated with sexual dysfunction exist for women including: individual general health status, diabetes mellitus, cardiovascular disease, psychiatric/psychological disorders, other chronic diseases, and socio-demographic conditions.

Muniyappa R, Norton M, Dunn ME, Banerji MA. Diabetes and female sexual dysfunction: moving beyond "benign neglect." Curr Diab Rep. 2005;5:230–6. Annotation: Diabetes may affect the female sexual response from desire to arousal and orgasm, but diabetes particularly affects arousal with decreased genital sensation and lubrication. Vaginal dryness and infections may lead to dyspareunia. Predictors of sexual dysfunction in women include depression, low androgens as well as possibly estrogens, which may be etiologic, in addition to numerous medications used by patients with diabetes. Practitioners should recognize the high prevalence of female sexual dysfunction, up to 50%.

Salonia A, Lanzi R, Scavini M, Pontillo M, Gatti E, Petrella G, Licata G, Nappi RE, Bosi E, Briganti A, Rigatti P, Montorsi F. Sexual function and endocrine profile in fertile women with type 1 diabetes. Diabetes Care. 2006;29:312–6. Annotation: Fifty fertile women with type 1 diabetes and 47 healthy control subjects participated. Among type 1 diabetic women, sexual function and sexual distress vary according to the phase of the menstrual cycle. During the luteal phase, type 1 diabetic women had decreased sexual function and increased sexual distress, compared with control subjects.

Hysterectomy

Hysterectomy, or surgical removal of the uterus, may be performed for treatment of cervical cancer. In a woman with cervical cancer, in addition to a total hysterectomy, adjacent lymph nodes and surrounding tissues containing nerves may also be removed. This kind of hysterectomy is called a radical hysterectomy. The uterus may be removed for treatment of non-cancerous growths, called fibroids, that sometimes cause heavy menstrual bleeding or severe menstrual cramps. The removal of the entire uterus is called a total hysterectomy. The uterus could be surgically removed, sparing the cervix, to preserve nerves in the region that pass to the vagina. This kind of hysterectomy is called a subtotal hysterectomy and is performed to maximize preservation of sexual function. Since important nerves that provide sensation pathways to and from the vagina pass near the cervix, it is postulated that nerve-sparing hysterectomy procedures be considered, especially in women who experience high sexual satisfaction with internal-based orgasms. During any procedure to remove the uterus, a decision is made to preserve or to remove the woman's ovaries. The argument is that removal of the ovaries prevents the possibility of ovarian cancer. After any kind of hysterectomy, with or without ovary removal, there may be changes in a woman's sexual function.

What do the studies reveal? As it concerns radical hysterectomy, Jensen and colleagues reported the results of the sexual function of women who underwent radical hysterectomy for treatment of early cervical cancer. Compared to an age-matched control group, women who underwent radical hysterectomy experienced significantly less sexual interest and decreased vaginal lubrication that persisted over several years of follow-up. On the other hand, other surgically-related sexual and vaginal problems associated with the radical hysterectomy, such as uncomfortable sexual intercourse due to a reduced vaginal size, decreased with time.

Carlson reported that in women undergoing total hysterectomy for non-cancerous conditions (excessive bleeding, cramps, pain) there was a marked improvement in symptoms and quality of life during the early years after surgery. Rhodes and colleagues also examined measures of sexual function in women undergoing total hysterectomy. These authors showed that both sexual desire and frequency of sexual relations significantly increased after hysterectomy and throughout the follow-up period. Similarly, frequency of orgasm significantly increased and strength of orgasm rose dramatically after hysterectomy.

As it concerns the difference between total hysterectomy and subtotal hysterectomy in terms of sparing sexual function, Gimbel and colleagues examined the sexual satisfaction of women undergoing either procedure for benign uterine conditions, such as fibroids. The authors reported that both groups had the same sexual satisfaction outcome. Zobbe and colleagues also studied the sexual outcome following total vs. subtotal hysterectomy for benign uterine conditions. The authors found no significant differences between the 2 hysterectomy procedures at the 1-year follow-up with regard to women's sexual desire, frequency of intercourse, frequency of orgasm, quality of orgasm, localization of orgasm, satisfaction with sexual life, and sexual pain. In both total and subtotal hysterectomy groups, there was a significant reduction in sexual pain.

Regarding the hormone status of women after hysterectomy, Cutler and colleagues measured the post-operative hormonal impact on women's sexual health and overall quality of life. The authors found that the combination of total hysterectomy and bilateral oophorectomy may worsen the clinical and quality of life picture. The authors stressed that the ovaries provide approximately half of a woman's testosterone and, after surgery, many women reported impaired sexual functioning, especially loss of sexual interest, despite estrogen treatment. Rako also reported on the important observation that the ovaries are a critical source of both estrogen and testosterone. Vaginal dryness, night sweats, and hot flashes are associated with the estrogen deficiency caused by bilateral oophorectomy (surgical menopause). Rako stated that, on removal of the uterus, even if the ovaries are spared, ovarian estrogen and testosterone function could be reduced. Rako noted that low testosterone values after a hysterectomy are associated with a decrease in sexual libido, sexual pleasure, and wellbeing.

In summary, it appears that for women with cervical cancer who undergo a radical hysterectomy, expectations are appropriate that changes in sexual function may result post-operatively. For women with severe clinical symptoms of fibroids, total or subtotal hysterectomy may actually result in improved sexual function. In women who undergo surgical menopause, the combination of a hysterectomy and bilateral ovary removal, hormone changes will occur, and this may be a basis for changes in sexual function. Research is needed regarding the value of surgically sparing, during hysterectomy, pelvic autonomic nerves that pass to and from the vagina. This type of surgery deserves consideration in an effort to improve quality of life.

References for Hysterectomy:

Dennerstein L, Koochaki P, Barton I, Graziottin A. Hypoactive sexual desire disorder in menopausal women: a survey of Western European women. J Sex Med. 2006;3:212–22. Annotation: A cross-sectional survey of 2,467 European women in France, Germany, Italy, and the United Kingdom was performed. A greater proportion of surgically menopausal women had low sexual desire, compared with pre-menopausal or naturally menopausal women. Surgically menopausal women were more likely to have hypoactive sexual desire disorder than pre-menopausal or naturally menopausal women. Sexual desire scores and sexual arousal, orgasm, and sexual pleasure were highly correlated, demonstrating that low sexual desire is frequently associated with decreased functioning in other aspects of sexual response. Women with low sexual desire were less likely to engage in sexual activity and more likely to be dissatisfied with their sex life and partner relationship than women with normal desire.

Dragisic KG, Milad MP. Sexual functioning and patient expectations of sexual functioning after hysterectomy. Am J Obstet Gynecol. 2004;190:1416–8. Annotation: A total of 75 patients who had undergone hysterectomy were surveyed about sexual function. Hysterectomy had no effect on the frequency of sexual activity or on orgasmic response. Post-operatively, patients were less likely to report pain with intercourse.

El-Toukhy TA, Hefni M, Davies A, Mahadevan S. The effect of different types of hysterectomy on urinary and sexual functions: a prospective study. J Obstet Gynaecol. 2004;24:420–5. Annotation: A prospective observational study was designed to evaluate the effect of the different techniques of hysterectomy on sexual function. A total of 184 women admitted for hysterectomy participated. Patients underwent one of four different techniques of hysterectomy. At 6 months after surgery, patients reported significantly lower rates of deep dyspareunia than before the operation, regardless of the hysterectomy technique used.

Ferroni P, Deeble J. Women's subjective experience of hysterectomy. Aust Health Rev. 1996;19:40–55. Annotation: A sample of 656 women completed a questionnaire, 107 of them having undergone hysterectomy. Few women regarded the uterus as "essential to femininity or womanhood," and very few saw it as affecting sexuality. Women in the hysterectomy group reported that their satisfaction with sexual activity had improved, whereas those who had a hysterectomy and concomitant gynecological conditions believed that it had deteriorated.

Flory N, Bissonnette F, Binik YM. Psychosocial effects of hysterectomy: literature review. J Psychosom Res. 2005;59:117–29. Annotation: Over 100 studies and reviews, in English, French, and German, published in the past 30 years regarding psychosocial effects of hysterectomy were examined. A range of 10%

to 20% of women reported negative outcomes, such as reduced sexual interest, arousal, and orgasm, as well as elevated depressive symptoms and impaired body image.

Flory N, Bissonnette F, Amsel RT, Binik YM. The psychosocial outcomes of total and subtotal hysterectomy: A randomized controlled trial. J Sex Med. 2006;3:483–91. Annotation: The 32 total hysterectomy (laparoscopic assisted vaginal hysterectomy) patients and the 31 supracervical laparoscopic hysterectomy patients experienced significant improvement in overall sexual functioning. For both groups, pain in the abdomen during gynecological examinations was significantly reduced.

Goetsch MF. The effect of total hysterectomy on specific sexual sensations. Am J Obstet Gynecol. 2005;192:1922–7. Annotation: A total of 105 women who underwent a total hysterectomy participated. Ease of sexual arousal diminished in 24% and improved in 11%. Intensity of orgasms decreased in 15% and increased in 14%. Sexual satisfaction increased significantly. Seven women noted distinctly worse sexual function.

Kuppermann M, Varner RE, Summitt RL Jr, Learman LA, Ireland C, Vittinghoff E, Stewart AL, Lin F, Richter HE, Showstack J, Hulley SB, Washington AE. Effect of hysterectomy vs medical treatment on health-related quality of life and sexual functioning: the medicine or surgery (Ms) randomized trial. JAMA. 2004;291:1447–55. Annotation: A total of 63 pre-menopausal women were randomly assigned to undergo hysterectomy or medical treatment. At 6 months, women in the hysterectomy group had greater improvement in symptom resolution and sexual desire.

Kuppermann M, Summitt RL Jr, Varner RE, McNeeley SG, Goodman-Gruen D, Learman LA, Ireland CC, Vittinghoff E, Lin F, Richter HE, Showstack J, Hulley SB, Washington AE. Sexual functioning after total compared with supracervical hysterectomy: a randomized trial. Obstet Gynecol. 2005;105:1309–18. Annotation: A total of 135 women underwent abdominal hysterectomy as a total or supracervical procedure. Sexual problems improved dramatically in both groups during the first 6 months and reached a plateau by 1 year. At 2 years, both groups reported few problems with sexual functioning, and there were no significant differences between groups.

Lowenstein L, Yarnitsky D, Gruenwald I, Deutsch M, Sprecher E, Gedalia U, Vardi Y. Does hysterectomy affect genital sensation? Eur J Obstet Gynecol Reprod Biol. 2005;119:242–5. Annotation: Twenty-seven women were admitted for elective hysterectomy. Genital sensation testing and sexual function information was obtained before and after the surgery. There was significant decrease in sensation to cold and warm stimuli at the anterior and posterior vaginal wall after surgery. Clitoral sensation remained unchanged after surgery. Despite the changed sensations, few reported any decline in sexual function. These findings highlight the importance of clitoral, as compared to vaginal, sensation in sexual function.

McPherson K, Herbert A, Judge A, Clarke A, Bridgman S, Maresh M, Overton C. Psychosexual health 5 years after hysterectomy: population-based comparison with endometrial ablation for dysfunctional uterine bleeding. Health Expect. 2005;8:234–43. Annotation: Over 8,900 women who underwent either transcervical endometrial resection/ablation or subtotal and total hysterectomy, with and without prophylactic bilateral oophorectomy, participated. Five years after surgery, the prevalence of sexual problems was higher after hysterectomy than after transcervical endometrial resection/ablation. Among the women with concurrent bilateral oophorectomy, libido loss increased by 80%, difficult sexual arousal increased by 82%, and vaginal dryness increased by 69%, compared with transcervical endometrial resection/ablation. Women should be advised that they might be at higher risk for sexual problems following hysterectomy, compared with a less invasive procedure.

Salonia A, Briganti A, Deho F, Zanni G, Rigatti P, Montorsi F. Women's sexual dysfunction: a review of the "surgical landscape". Eur Urol. 2006;50:44-52. Annotation: Studies were analyzed that provided any functional outcome data about urogynecologic surgery, such as hysterectomy. Urogynecologic or oncologic pelvic surgery may have a significant impact on women's sexual health. Data about the functional outcome after hysterectomy are often contradictory, and more clinical trials are needed.

Vomvolaki E, Kalmantis K, Kioses E, Antsaklis A. The effect of hysterectomy on sexuality and psychological changes. Eur J Contracept Reprod Health Care. 2006;11:23–7. Annotation: Studies published in different journals were compared. Women are more likely to report improved sexual functioning after surgery when their symptoms have been alleviated. A new hysterectomy procedure that "spares" abdominal ligaments and nerves is quicker, resulting in less blood loss and shorter hospital stays, seeming to respect the tissues more, without affecting the sexuality of the women.

Walker WJ, Barton-Smith P. Long-term follow up of uterine artery embolization—an effective alternative in the treatment of fibroids. BJOG. 2006;113:464–8. Annotation: A total of 258 women were identified as being 5–7 years post-uterine artery embolization for treatment of symptomatic uterine fibroids. Based on responses to a questionnaire, more than 80% of fibroid-related symptoms were still resolved or improved. Premature menopause directly following uterine artery embolization occurred in only one woman in the study group. A total of 88% of women were satisfied with the outcome of the procedure at 5–7 years and would choose it again or recommend it to others.

Male Partner's Sexual Health

Couples share their sexual dysfunctions. Can a woman develop a sexual dysfunction exclusively because of her partner's sexual problem? There are limited scientific data on the topic. Based on the information available, the answer is probably yes. The data are less clear for women without sexual dysfunction who have women partners with sexual dysfunction, however women who are with men with erectile dysfunction or premature ejaculation may indeed have their own sexual function adversely affected.

Erectile dysfunction was the most frequently cited reason for cessation of sexual activity in a sample of over 500 otherwise healthy women. In another study, the sexual function was compared between almost 40 women whose men had erectile dysfunction and almost 50 women whose men did not. Women's sexual arousal, lubrication, orgasm, satisfaction, and pain were significantly diminished among women with men who had erectile dysfunction in comparison to women in the control group.

An additional study was performed on almost 300 women in 8 countries whose male partners had erectile dysfunction. Women whose partners had erectile dysfunction reported a lower frequency of sexual activity currently, compared with before their partner developed erectile difficulties. Significantly fewer women reported that they experienced "almost always" or "most times" sexual desire, sexual arousal, orgasm or sexual satisfaction currently, compared with before their partners developed erectile difficulties. In addition, women had the lowest frequency of orgasm and the lowest satisfaction with sexual experience when their male partners had the severest form of erectile dysfunction. Women whose partners were current users of phosphodiesterase type 5 inhibitor therapy, e.g., sildenafil, reported significantly greater frequency of desire, arousal, and orgasm than did women whose partners were not current phosphodiesterase type 5 inhibitor users.

Further, a trial was performed in women whose male partners had erectile dysfunction but the female partner did *not* have sexual dysfunction. Compared to the women whose men with erectile dysfunction were treated with placebo, women whose partners were randomized to receive the active drug had significantly higher sexual quality of life, sexual desire, arousal, lubrication, orgasm, and satisfaction. Women's sexual function improvements correlated with treatment related improvements of their partner's erectile function. Clinical management of sexual dysfunctions should emphasize both members of the couple.

Another erectile problem men suffer from is Peyronie's disease, which is characterized by a hard lump or plaque that forms on the surface of the erection chamber lining, deep under the skin. Peyronie's disease symptoms include penile pain during erection, penile curvature and loss of penile length during erection, and erectile dysfunction. Peyronie's disease may be related to the female partner superior position sexual activity. If the female partner misses with her penetration and brings her body weight to bear on the penile erection, the excessive force borne to the erection causes localized inflammation and injury to the tunica. In some cases, this can lead to tunica inflammation, with subsequent scarring eventually causing penile curvature during erection. The bend in the penis may make sexual intercourse penetration difficult, or may cause pain to the partner upon penetration.

Premature ejaculation is a very common male sexual dysfunction, affecting approximately 25% of men. Premature ejaculation may be objectively determined using a stopwatch to record intravaginal ejaculatory latency time, defined as the time between vaginal intromission and intravaginal ejaculation. It has been suggested that an intravaginal ejaculatory latency time of 2 minutes or less may serve as a criterion for defining premature ejaculation.

One study compared the mean intravaginal ejaculatory latency time of 200 men with premature ejaculation to almost 1400 men without premature ejaculation. The intravaginal ejaculatory latency time was 1.8 minutes in the former and 7.3 minutes in the latter. Women whose men had premature ejaculation were found to significantly differ from women whose men did not have premature ejaculation, in terms of decreased satisfaction with sexual intercourse and increased interpersonal difficulty and distress.

In summary, couples' sexual problems and sexual solutions are shared. There are data documenting that women, whose male partners have erectile dysfunction and/or premature ejaculation, can develop their own sexual dysfunction based on their male partners' sexual problems.

What can be done about your male partner's sexual dysfunction? There are many FDA-approved treatment options for men with erectile dysfunction. Erectile dysfunction is the persistent or repeated inability, for at least 3 months duration, to attain and/or maintain an erection sufficient for satisfactory sexual performance. It is a significant and common medical problem. If your partner has erectile dysfunction, he should see a healthcare professional and, if needed, a sexual medicine specialist.

What should you and your male partner do about his erectile dysfunction? He should undergo a comprehensive medical and psychosexual history, physical examination, and laboratory testing, just as is required for a woman being treated for sexual health problems. Laboratory tests may include sex steroid hormones, blood flow or genital sensation testing. Your partner may need exercise testing to see if there are any early signs of blockage in other arteries, such as in the heart. He may need to change his diet and consider a Mediterranean diet. He may need to start a daily exercise program and consider stopping smoking. He may need counseling with you to address relationship factors, such as excessive marital tension. The sexual health problem should be characterized, and the need for additional testing and referral assessed. Your partner's needs and your needs as a member of the couple, both your expectations and your priorities, are key elements in the management process. Healthcare providers in general, and specifically sexual medicine healthcare providers, can offer evidence-based treatment options if your partner has erectile dysfunction.

Sex therapy may be provided to your partner alone or ideally with both you and your partner as a couple. Sex therapy addresses specific psychological or interpersonal factors that are likely to enhance your partner's and your sexual functioning. Factors that frequently interfere with sexual satisfaction are relationship distress, sexual performance concerns, and dysfunctional communication patterns. Independent, brief sex therapy consists of in-session discussion and at-home exercises specific for your partner and for your couple relationship. Cognitive-behavioral interventions are used predominantly, and include such strategies as behavioral rehearsal, cognitive restructuring/reframing, systematic sensitization, anger management, thought stopping techniques, control and perception of control, self-esteem enhancement, goal setting, active listening, strategies for coping with stress, and modification of life-style, such as getting better sleep, better nutrition, and more exercise. Sex therapy can be used in conjunction with oral phosphodiesterase type 5 inhibitors, constriction devices or other medical/surgical treatments. This modified form of sex therapy can address the psychological reactions to the medical treatment, which may be perceived as an unnatural or unacceptable means of achieving sexual gratification.

Oral phosphodiesterase type 5 inhibitors are FDA approved for the treatment of erectile dysfunction. They are administered on demand, in appropriate dosages, and are effective in facilitating the initiation and maintenance of erections following sexual stimulation approximately 30–45 minutes after administration. No notable effects on erections are observed in the absence of sexual stimulation. Phosphodiesterase type 5 inhibitors are effective across a broad range of causes of erectile dysfunction, including psychologic, medication-related, vascular, and neurologic. Side effects include headaches, flushing, upset stomach, nasal congestion, and back or leg pain. Phosphodiesterase type 5 inhibitors are contraindicated for men receiving nitrate therapy, including short or long acting agents, delivered by oral, sublingual, transnasal or topical administration.

Vacuum constriction device therapy is a well-established, non invasive therapy that is FDA approved for over-the-counter distribution. Vacuum constriction device therapy may represent an attractive treatment alternative if your male partner does not desire the use of medications, such as oral phosphodiesterase type 5 inhibitors. The vacuum constriction device applies a negative pressure to your partner's penis thus drawing in blood. The blood is then retained by the application of an elastic constriction band at the base of the penis. The side effects associated with vacuum device therapy include penile pain, numbness, bruising, and delayed ejaculation.

Testosterone therapy should be pursued, especially if your partner has consistently low values of "unbound" testosterone documented on repeated blood testing. The "calculated free testosterone" values, as determined by measuring the total testosterone, the sex hormone binding globulin, and the albumin levels, should be higher than 5 ng/dl. The syndrome of low biologically available testosterone, with symptoms such as fatigue or low interest, is called hypogonadism or androgen insufficiency. The most common form of testosterone therapy is by topical delivery of an FDA approved gel, although testosterone may be administered by intramuscular injection. Testosterone therapy should be used selectively and carefully. Your male partner will need to undergo a digital rectal examination and a blood test called "PSA" or prostate specific antigen prior to any testosterone therapy. It is contraindicated to administer testosterone to a man with prostate cancer, as the testosterone can encourage the growth of a pre-existing prostate cancer. If the rectal examination and the PSA blood tests are initially normal, your male partner will need to have repeated examinations and blood tests during regular follow-up visits while on testosterone therapy. Often, giving testosterone therapy will improve the effects of the phosphodiesterase type 5 inhibitors in facilitating, initiating, and maintaining erections, although this effect takes months to be appreciated.

Intraurethral administration of alprostadil is another FDA approved therapy option for erectile dysfunction. The alprostadil is in the form of a semi-solid pellet that is placed in the male urethra with a special inserter device, prior to sexual activity. Approximately 50% of men achieve successful intercourse with this system in the home situation. Side effects associated with the intraurethral administration of alprostadil include penile pain and, more uncommonly, prolonged erections. In addition to local side effects, intraurethral alprostadil may cause systemic effects, particularly hypotension, in a small number of cases.

Penile self-injection therapy uses the FDA approved drug prostaglandin E_1. The drug is injected directly into the side of the penis into the erection chamber, prior to sexual activity, with a small gauge insulin-like needle and syringe. If your partner needs this therapy, he will need to be trained by a healthcare provider as to the correct techniques for self-administration. Often, the woman injects the penis if the man is unable to do this. Penile self-injection therapy is remarkably effective in most cases of biologically-based erectile dysfunction. In general, penile self-injection therapy with alprostadil is effective in 70% to 80% of patients, although discontinuation rates are very high in most studies. In addition to prostaglandin E_1 therapy, various combinations of prostaglandin E_1, phentolamine, and/or papaverine are widely used for self-injection therapy. Side effects of penile self-injection therapy include primarily local penile events, such as prolonged erections or priapism (<1%) and pain (5% to 20%), as well as scar tissue formation with chronic use. Penile self-injection therapy should not be used if your partner is receiving the anti-depressant medication monoamine oxidase inhibitor. Penile self-injection therapy continues to be widely used and is a safe and effective non-surgical treatment for erectile dysfunction, especially when simpler, less invasive treatments are either not effective or not indicated.

Surgical implantation of a semi-rigid or inflatable penile prosthesis is highly invasive and associated with potential complications, such as infection in 1% to 5% of cases or mechanical failure. Penile prosthesis insertion is an irreversible treatment option, generally reserved for select cases of severe, treatment-refractory erectile dysfunction, such as Peyronie's Disease, priapism or after radical prostatectomy. Despite the invasiveness, numerous studies have shown penile prostheses to be associated with high rates of sexual satisfaction for both partners. The inflatable penile prosthesis provides a more aesthetic erection and better concealment than the semi-rigid prosthesis. Penile prostheses provide an effective surgical solution for erectile dysfunction, particularly in those patients for whom other forms of therapy are ineffective.

Penile microsurgical revascularization surgery may correct erectile dysfunction, particularly in young men (aged < 40–45 years) with a history of pelvic and/or perineal trauma, such as from a fall onto a bicycle bar or kick in the crotch. If a localized arterial blockage is determined to exist, a revascularization procedure employing a new artery source (e.g., the inferior epigastric artery) to deliver blood to the erection artery of the penis is a treatment option. Penile revascularization is associated with a 60% to 70% long-term (5-year) success rate and few complications.

What if your male partner has premature ejaculation? While there are no FDA approved treatments for premature ejaculation at this time, most healthcare providers or sexual medicine specialists will use the following treatment options alone or in combination. First, a desensitizing agent such as topical lidocaine is used to reduce penile sensation. Usually the desensitizing agent is applied in conjunction with a condom, to avoid drug transfer to the woman's genital tissues. It is important to see if the desensitizing agent used may adversely affect the integrity of the condom, if contraception is important. The idea is that less penile sensation will lower the likelihood of premature ejaculation. Second, an anti-depressant that is a selective serotonin reuptake inhibitor is used daily. At present there are no selective serotonin reuptake inhibitors FDA approved for the treatment of premature ejaculation. There are many different selective serotonin reuptake inhibitors available for treatment of depression, most of which can be used off-label for premature ejaculation. The idea is that serotonin is a specific centrally acting inhibitor of sexual activity, especially ejaculation and orgasm. Correct daily dosing of the selective serotonin reuptake inhibitor can increase the intravaginal ejaculatory latency time. Third, an oral phosphodiesterase type 5 inhibitor can be used. The idea is that if your partner has an early ejaculation, he will be able to obtain a second erection earlier by using a phosphodiesterase type 5 inhibitor. As a last treatment option, penile self-injection therapy may be used, resulting in an erection that will last post-ejaculation. As in all cases of sexual dysfunction, consultation with a sexual medicine specialist may be needed.

In summary, sexual problems and sexual solutions are shared. Management of sexual health problems requires the use of evidence-based, rational, clear, and specific guidelines for diagnosing and treating men and women with sexual health problems. The treatment of a sexual dysfunction in one partner may heighten the awareness of a sexual health issue in the other. Both you and your partner should undergo general medical and psychosocial evaluation by a healthcare provider or by a sexual medicine specialist at regular intervals. Follow up is intended to assess the progress of current therapy. A sound and trusting relationship among you, your partner, and your healthcare provider is the key to success in a sexual medicine treatment program. Sexual health is an important element in the physical and psychological wellbeing of most individuals and couples.

References for Male Partner's Sexual Health:

Althof SE, Turner LA, Levine SB, Bodner D, Kursh ED, Resnick MI. Through the eyes of women: the sexual and psychological responses of women to their partner's treatment with self-injection or external vacuum therapy. J Urol. 1992;147:1024–7. Annotation: Sexual, marital, and psychological responses of women to their male partner's use of erectile dysfunction treatments were evaluated. Women partners demonstrated significant increases in frequency of intercourse, sexual arousal, coital orgasm, and sexual satisfaction. Women partners reported feeling more at ease in their relationships and characterized sex as more leisurely, relaxed, and assured. Self-injection and vacuum pump therapy secondarily facilitate improved sexual function in women.

Althof SE, Eid JF, Talley DR, Brock GB, Dunn ME, Tomlin ME, Natanegara F, Ahuja S. Through the eyes of women: the partners' perspective on tadalafil. Urology. 2006;68:631–5. Annotation: A total of 746 couples, (men with erectile dysfunction and the untreated partner) were randomized to placebo or tadalafil. Tadalafil significantly improved the responses for a partner-evaluated sexual satisfaction questionnaire. Partners tended to report greater overall satisfaction than patients at baseline and post-baseline. For successful intercourse attempts, partners treated with tadalafil reported more overall satisfaction than those treated with placebo.

Cayan S, Bozlu M, Canpolat B, Akbay E. The assessment of sexual functions in women with male partners complaining of erectile dysfunction: does treatment of male sexual dysfunction improve female partner's sexual functions? J Sex Marital Ther. 2004;30:333–41. Annotation: The study included 38 women with male partners complaining of erectile dysfunction (ED) and 49 women with male partners who did not have ED. Sexual arousal, lubrication, orgasm, satisfaction, pain, and total score were significantly lower in the women with male partners complaining of ED than in the control group. After the treatment of male ED, significant improvement in sexual arousal, lubrication, orgasm, satisfaction, and pain was observed in the women.

Fisher WA, Rosen RC, Eardley I, Sand M, Goldstein I. Sexual experience of female partners of men with erectile dysfunction: the female experience of men's attitudes to life events and sexuality (FEMALES) study. J Sex Med. 2005;2:675–84. Annotation: A total of 293 female partners of men with ED responded to questionnaires. After their partner developed ED in comparison with before, women reported engaging in sexual activity significantly less frequently. Significantly fewer women experienced sexual desire, arousal or orgasm "almost always" or "most times," and significantly fewer women reported satisfaction with their sexual relationship after their partner developed ED compared with before. Decreases in female sexual satisfaction and frequency of orgasm were significantly related to the male partner's self-reported severity of ED. The proportion of women who experienced sexual desire, arousal, and orgasm "almost always" or "most times" was significantly higher in the group whose partners were currently using a PDE5 inhibitor.

Fisher WA, Rosen RC, Mollen M, Brock G, Karlin G, Pommerville P, Goldstein I, Bangerter K, Bandel TJ, Derogatis LR, Sand M. Improving the sexual quality of life of couples affected by erectile dysfunction: a double-blind, randomized, placebo-controlled trial of vardenafil. J Sex Med. 2005;2:699–708. Annotation: This was a randomized, double-blind, multi-center, flexible-dose, parallel-group comparison of vardenafil vs. placebo for 12 weeks in men with ED and their female partners. Compared with placebo, vardenafil significantly improved the female partner's response to the quality of life domain of the modified Sexual Life Quality Questionnaire.

Goldstein I, Fisher WA, Sand M, Rosen RC, Mollen M, Brock G, Karlin G, Pommerville P, Bangerter K, Bandel TJ, Derogatis LR. Women's sexual function improves when partners are administered vardenafil for erectile dysfunction: a prospective, randomized, double-blind, placebo-controlled trial. J Sex Med. 2005;2:819–32. Annotation: A randomized, double-blind, placebo-controlled, multi-institutional comparison of vardenafil versus placebo was performed in 229 couples, consisting of the treated man with ED and the untreated woman partner. Compared with placebo, in the untreated woman partner, vardenafil significantly increased the Sexual Life Quality Questionnaire, the total Female Sexual Function Index, and sexual desire, subjective arousal, lubrication, orgasm, and satisfaction domains. Treatment-related improvement in erectile function was correlated reliably with improvement in women partners' Female Sexual Function Index total and individual domain scores.

Kizilkaya Beji N, Yalcin O, Ayyildiz EH, Kayir A. Effect of urinary leakage on sexual function during sexual intercourse. Urol Int. 2005;74:250–5. Annotation: This study examined 32 incontinent women with urinary leakage during sexual intercourse and a control group of 60 women without urinary leakage. The women with urinary incontinence were 4.7 times less satisfied with their sexual life and their partners had ejaculation without full erection 3.1 times more. Urinary leakage during coitus affects women's and men's sex life adversely.

Rosen R, Janssen E, Wiegel M, Bancroft J, Althof S, Wincze J, Segraves RT, Barlow D. Psychological and interpersonal correlates in men with erectile dysfunction and their partners: a pilot study of treatment outcome with sildenafil. J Sex Marital Ther. 2006;32:215–34. Annotation: Sixty-nine men with ED and their partners were enrolled in a sildenafil treatment trial. Significant improvements were seen in partners' ratings of sexual function including arousal, pleasure, and orgasm.

Shindel A, Quayle S, Yan Y, Husain A, Naughton C. Sexual dysfunction in female partners of men who have undergone radical prostatectomy correlates with sexual dysfunction of the male partner. J Sex Med. 2005;2:833–41. Annotation: Ninety couples participated in this retrospective study to assess sexuality in the female partners of men who have undergone radical prostatectomy for prostate cancer. Female Sexual Function Index domain scores correlated with

International Index of Erectile Function domain scores, indicating an interrelationship between male and female sexual dysfunction in these couples. Evaluation and treatment of sexual dysfunction after radical prostatectomy should involve both partners.

Turner LA, Althof SE, Levine SB, Tobias TR, Kursh ED, Bodner D, Resnick MI. Treating erectile dysfunction with external vacuum devices: impact upon sexual, psychological and marital functioning. J Urol. 1990;144:79-82. Annotation: A total of 18 female partners of men who used external vacuum devices in the treatment of erectile dysfunction participated. These women reported improved sexual functioning, including increased frequency of orgasm, decreased masturbation, and greater sexual satisfaction.

Menopause

Menopause is a natural biological process that consists of physical and psychosocial changes. This transition usually begins in a woman's early 40's, lasting into her 50's and, rarely, her 60's. The average age of menopause is 51, and is usually about two years earlier for smokers than non-smokers. Peri-menopause, when a woman still has her period, is the time when she may begin to experience menopausal signs and symptoms even though she is still ovulating. Menopause is considered to be the 12 months after a woman's last period. The years that follow are called post-menopause. Today, a woman may live as much as half of her life after menopause.

What causes menopause? During reproductive years, estrogen and progesterone levels vary and regulate monthly cycles of ovulation and menstruation. Menopause begins naturally when ovaries begin to make less estrogen and less progesterone. At menopause the ovaries cease estradiol synthesis, but may continue to make androgens during post-menopause. Menopause is usually a natural process, however certain treatments can initiate it. An operation that removes both uterus and ovaries (total hysterectomy and bilateral oophorectomy) causes "surgical menopause." With surgical menopause, there is no peri-menopausal phase. Chemotherapy and radiation therapy can also induce menopause. Premature ovarian failure is a rare cause of menopause, and may result from genetic factors or auto-immune disease.

Menopausal symptoms are different for each individual; women may experience any number of physical and emotional changes. The ten most common symptoms in no specific order include: irregular and unpredictable periods; vaginal burning, itching, atrophy or recurrent vaginal infections; urinary urgency, frequency, recurrent urinary tract infections or urinary incontinence; hot flashes, night or day sweats, chills, facial flushing or skin erythema on the chest, neck, and arms; sleep disturbances, sleep deprivation, tiredness or fatigue that may affect your mood and overall health; changes in appearance such as weight gain, especially in fat above your waist and abdomen, loss of fullness in your breasts, thinning hair, wrinkles, coarse hair on your chin, upper lip, chest, and abdomen; irritability and increased stress due to life events such as the illness or death of a parent, adult child's departure from home or return to home or retirement; decreased memory and diminished concentration; coronary heart disease, osteoporotic fractures or other new medical problems; and diminished sexual interest, diminished sexual arousal including vaginal dryness, thinning of the vaginal wall, diminished lubrication, diminished intensity of orgasm, dyspareunia or painful intercourse.

Women in the peri-menopausal and post-menopausal years frequently encounter sexual health problems. During peri- and post-menopause, compared to pre-menopause, sexual health problems occur more frequently, are more often irreversible, and are more likely to be progressive, particularly if the cause is associated with vaginal atrophy secondary to estrogen deficiency.

Why do sexual problems occur during the peri-menopause and menopause? Officially, menopause occurs when the ovaries cease making estradiol. Estradiol is a very important hormone that helps facilitate the woman's sexual response. In some menopausal women, estradiol can still be naturally synthesized. This, however, does not occur in the ovary but through conversion of androgens to estrogens in the adrenal gland or in the periphery such as fat tissue. If the estradiol values are adequate, some women may not experience many signs and symptoms of menopause.

How important is estradiol to genital tissues? Simply stated, estrogens are very critical for normal genital tissue structure and function. Diminished estrogen production may render your genital tissues susceptible to atrophy within weeks to months. Vaginal atrophy secondary to low estradiol is a key contributor to post-menopausal sexual health problems. In an estrogen-rich environment, the normal vaginal flora keep the vaginal pH in the acid range and discourage growth of certain bacteria and yeast. In post-menopausal women, the pH becomes neutral or alkaline. This increases the likelihood of vaginal discharge and odor.

What is vaginal atrophy? Atrophy of the vagina may cause it to become pale or colorless. There is loss of the multiple folds that are present in the estrogenized vagina allowing it to stretch and widen during sexual arousal. Atrophy of the blood vessel layer of the vagina may cause diminished blood flow, resulting in decreased lubrication and vaginal dryness. Thinning of the vaginal lining layer may cause it to bleed. When intercourse is attempted under conditions of low estradiol, sexual activity can be painful, unpleasant, and unsatisfactory.

There are many ways in which low estradiol adversely affects genital tissues. Estrogen deficiency may result in reduced genital sensation. The clitoral hood may become scarred. The glans clitoris may atrophy. There may be thinning of the hair of the mons and atrophy and shrinkage of the labia minora and labia majora with decreased subcutaneous fat and skin elasticity. Low estradiol may prolong the time to achieving genital vasocongestion or arousal. There may also be reduced intensity and number of vaginal and uterine contractions during orgasm.

In addition to estrogens, androgens are also critical in maintaining genital tissue structure and function in menopausal women. Androgens also improve desire and orgasm responses, bone and skeletal muscle metabolism, cognition, feelings of wellbeing, and mood. It is important to measure and, if appropriate, manage both estrogen and androgen hormones in the post-menopause. In summary, low estradiol and androgen levels may adversely affect sexual health. The low frequency of sexual activity can in turn lead to a vicious cycle of avoidance, performance anxiety, and decreased sexual desire.

Although sexual concerns are common, many post-menopausal women do not discuss the subject with healthcare providers. Some peri-menopausal and post-menopausal women believe their sexual function is too personal and too private to discuss even when they are bothered by a sexual health problem. For some women, their quality of life may not be negatively impacted by sexual problems. However, for other women, sexual health issues can be associated with significant personal distress and may result in lowered self-esteem, as well as a significant reduction in life satisfaction and quality of the couple's relationship. If you are distressed by your sexual health problems, you should talk with your healthcare provider concerning treatment of sexual health concerns.

What treatments are available? Do you have to use hormones? Prior to initiating any hormonal intervention, treatments may involve modification of reversible causes. These would include sex therapy, couples' counseling, lifestyle modification, dietary changes, increase in daily exercise, use of vaginal lubricants, medication changes, and use of vibrators or vacuum clitoris therapy devices. Hormonal therapy, local and/or systemic, may be eventually indicated, but a full disclosure of risks and benefits needs to be provided.

The take home message is that your sexual response is a complex, interactive process involving a unique set of mind, body, and partner issues. It is important to understand that successful treatment of vaginal atrophy with hormones may NOT correct dyspareunia, low interest, diminished arousal or muted orgasm if the woman being treated has psychosocial issues such as depression, is living with a violent partner or is the primary caregiver to a child with a chronic medical condition. All contributors to sexual health, not only hormonal ones, should be evaluated when considering treatment for peri-or post-menopausal sexual health problems.

References for Menopause:

Addis IB, Ireland CC, Vittinghoff E, Lin F, Stuenkel CA, Hulley S. Sexual activity and function in postmenopausal women with heart disease. Obstet Gynecol.

2005;106:121–7. Annotation: A total of 2,763 post-menopausal women, average age 67 years, with coronary disease and intact uteri participated. Approximately 39% of the women were sexually active, and 65% of these reported at least 1 of 5 sexual problems including lack of interest, inability to relax, difficulty in arousal or in orgasm, and discomfort with sex. Factors associated with being sexually active included: younger age, fewer years since menopause, being married, better self-reported health, not smoking, lack of chest discomfort, and not being depressed.

Avis NE, Zhao X, Johannes CB, Ory M, Brockwell S, Greendale GA. Correlates of sexual function among multi-ethnic middle-aged women: results from the Study of Women's Health Across the Nation (SWAN). Menopause. 2005;12:385–98. Annotation: Sexual function was studied in 3,167 non-Hispanic white, African American, Hispanic, Chinese, and Japanese women, 42–52 years old, pre- or early peri-menopausal, and not using hormones. Early peri-menopausal women reported significantly greater pain with intercourse than pre-menopausal women. Significant ethnic differences were found for arousal, pain, desire, and frequency of sexual intercourse. African American women reported higher frequency of sexual intercourse than white women. Hispanic women reported lower physical pleasure and arousal. Chinese women reported more pain and less desire and arousal than white women.

Davis SR, van der Mooren MJ, van Lunsen RH, Lopes P, Ribot J, Rees M, Moufarege A, Rodenberg C, Buch A, Purdie DW. Efficacy and safety of a testosterone patch for the treatment of hypoactive sexual desire disorder in surgically menopausal women: a randomized, placebo-controlled trial. Menopause. 2006;13:387–96. Annotation: A total of 61 surgically menopausal women receiving concurrent transdermal estrogen after oophorectomy who also had hypoactive sexual desire disorder participated. The testosterone-treated group experienced a significantly greater change from baseline in the domain sexual desire score compared with placebo. The domain scores for arousal, orgasm, decreased sexual concerns, responsiveness, and self-image, as well as decreased distress, were also significantly greater with testosterone therapy than placebo. Adverse events occurred with similar frequency in both groups, and no serious risks of therapy were observed.

Dennerstein L, Lehert P. Women's sexual functioning, lifestyle, mid-age, and menopause in 12 European countries. Menopause. 2004;11:778–85. Annotation: A total of 601 women aged 45–60 years consulted general practitioners in 12 European countries. The frequency of sexual intercourse varied significantly between countries, the highest being for the group of Latin or southern countries (France, Portugal, Italy, Spain). Change of partner, existence of partner, wellbeing, parity, and exercise were associated with both sexual response and frequency of sexual intercourse. Menopause status and stress were significantly associated with sexual response. Body mass index was significantly associated with frequency of sexual intercourse.

Dennerstein L, Lehert P, Burger H. The relative effects of hormones and relationship factors on sexual function of women through the natural menopausal transition. Fertil Steril. 2005;84:174–80. Annotation: A total of 336 Australian-born women aged 45–55 years who were still menstruating at baseline had 8 years of longitudinal data available for analysis. Prior level of sexual function, change in partner sexual function status, feelings for partner, and estradiol level predicted sexual response.

Dennerstein L, Hayes RD. Confronting the challenges: epidemiological study of female sexual dysfunction and the menopause. J Sex Med. 2005;2:S118–32. Annotation: It is possible to reach some tentative conclusions about how women's sexual function changes after menopause: post-menopausal women report a relatively high rate of sexual dysfunction (higher than men). There is a marked decline in sexual interest and frequency of sexual activity. This decline can be ameliorated by a number of psychosocial factors, although vaginal dryness and dyspareunia seem to be driven primarily by declining estradiol. The effects of menopause appear to be incremental and additional to those characteristics of aging.

Dennerstein L, Koochaki P, Barton I, Graziottin A. Hypoactive sexual desire disorder in menopausal women: a survey of Western European women. J Sex Med. 2006;3:212–22. Annotation: A total of 2,467 European women aged 20–70 years, residing in France, Germany, Italy, and the United Kingdom, participated. Surgically menopausal women were significantly more likely to have hypoactive sexual desire disorder than pre-menopausal or naturally menopausal women. Sexual desire scores and sexual arousal, orgasm, and sexual pleasure were highly correlated, demonstrating that low sexual desire is frequently associated with decreased functioning in other aspects of sexual response. Women with low sexual desire were less likely to engage in sexual activity and more likely to be dissatisfied with their sex life and partner relationship than women with normal desire.

Dennerstein L, Lehert P, Guthrie JR, Burger HG. Modeling women's health during the menopausal transition: a longitudinal analysis. Menopause. 2006; PMID:17023873. Annotation: A total of 336 Australian-born women participated, aged 45–55 years at baseline, who had menstruated in the prior 3 months. Declining levels of estradiol during the menopausal transition affected certain health outcomes: vasomotor symptoms, vaginal dryness, and sexual response. Wellbeing was negatively affected by stress. Exercise has beneficial effects on wellbeing. Relationship factors and mood affect sexual response.

Goldstein I, Alexander JL. Practical aspects in the management of vaginal atrophy and sexual dysfunction in perimenopausal and postmenopausal women. J Sex Med. 2005;2:S154–65. Annotation: The decline in circulating estrogen levels in peri- and post-menopause is associated with atrophy of tissues in the urogenital tract, and vaginal atrophy is an important contributor to post-menopausal sexual dysfunction. Estrogen decline disrupts many physiological responses characteristic of sexual arousal, including smooth muscle relaxation, vasocongestion, and vaginal lubrication; genital tissues depend on continued estrogen and androgen stimulation for normal function. An upward shift in vaginal pH as the result of vaginal atrophy alters the normal vaginal flora. Reduced lubrication capability and reduced tissue elasticity, in addition to shortening and narrowing of the vaginal vault, can lead to painful and/or unpleasant intercourse. At the same time, diminished sensory response may reduce orgasmic intensity. Other contributors to peri- and post-menopausal sexual dysfunction include reduced androgen levels, aging of multiple body systems, and side effects of medications. Clinical management includes measures to preserve and enhance overall health, adjustment of medication regimes to reduce or avoid side effects, and topical or systemic hormone supplementation with estrogens and/or androgens.

Graziottin A, Basson R. Sexual dysfunction in women with premature menopause. Menopause. 2004;11:766–77. Annotation: Premature menopause and loss of ovarian function in adolescence has several unique features concerning sexual health. Psychosexual maturity may be delayed. Maternity becomes ovodonation dependent. Sexual identity, sexual function, and sexual relationship are affected. Long-term safety data of estrogen and androgen therapies are minimal.

Graziottin A, Leiblum SR. Biological and psychosocial pathophysiology of female sexual dysfunction during the menopausal transition. J Sex Med. 2005;2:S133–45. Annotation: In menopause, the primary biological change is a decrease in circulating estrogen levels. Estrogen deficiency accounts for diminished vaginal lubrication. Continual estrogen loss is associated with changes in the vascular, muscular, and urogenital systems, and also alterations in mood, sleep, and cognitive functioning, all influencing sexual health. The age-dependent decline in testosterone may exacerbate aspects of female sexual dysfunction; these effects are most pronounced following bilateral oophorectomy. Physical and psychosexual changes may contribute to lower self-esteem, and diminished sexual responsiveness and sexual desire. Non-hormonal factors that affect sexuality are health status and current medication use, changes in or dissatisfaction with partner, partner's health and/or sexual problems, and socioeconomic status.

Jeong GW, Park K, Youn G, Kang HK, Kim HJ, Seo JJ, Ryu SB. Assessment of cerebrocortical regions associated with sexual arousal in premenopausal and menopausal women by using BOLD-based functional MRI. J Sex Med. 2005;2:645–51. Annotation: A total of 10 pre-menopausal and 10 menopausal women participated. The overall activated brain regions associated with sexual response of the pre-menopausal women were greater than those of the menopausal women. The limbic, temporal association areas, and parietal lobe showed greater enhancement of brain activation in pre-menopausal women. However, signal enhancement in the genu of the corpus callosum and superior frontal gyrus was dominant in menopausal women.

Leiblum S, Symonds T, Moore J, Soni P, Steinberg S, Sisson M. A methodology study to develop and validate a screener for hypoactive sexual desire disorder in postmenopausal women. J Sex Med. 2006;3:455–64. Annotation: A brief hypoactive sexual desire disorder screening tool was developed consisting of four self-report questions with an interpretable cut-score and concise confirmatory physician interview. Accuracy of the hypoactive sexual desire disorder screening tool was tested against in-depth interview diagnosis. The hypoactive sexual desire disorder screener can reliably detect the likely presence of hypoactive sexual desire disorder in post-menopausal women.

Madalinska JB, van Beurden M, Bleiker EM, Valdimarsdottir HB, Hollenstein J, Massuger LF, Gaarenstroom KN, Mourits MJ, Verheijen RH, van Dorst EB, van der Putten H, van der Velden K, Boonstra H, Aaronson NK. The impact of hormone replacement therapy on menopausal symptoms in younger high-risk women after prophylactic salpingo-oophorectomy. J Clin Oncol. 2006;24:3576–82. Annotation: A total of 450 pre-menopausal women at increased hereditary risk of ovarian cancer participated in this study. Compared with women in the repeated gynecologic screening group, oophorectomized hormone therapy users reported significantly more sexual discomfort due to vaginal dryness and dyspareunia.

Nappi RE, Wawra K, Schmitt S. Hypoactive sexual desire disorder in postmenopausal women. Gynecol Endocrinol. 2006;22:318–23. Annotation: Several recent, large studies have shown that the addition of transdermal testosterone to conventional estrogen/progestin hormone therapy can be helpful in surgically menopausal women presenting with hypoactive sexual desire disorder. After 24 weeks of treatment in these studies, testosterone-treated women experienced significantly greater increases in satisfying sexual activity and sexual desire, and greater decreases in distress, than placebo-treated women.

Sarrel PM. Androgen deficiency: menopause and estrogen-related factors. Fertil Steril. 2002;77 (Suppl 4):S63-7. Annotation: In menopausal women, the effects of estradiol depletion and replacement on sex hormone binding globulin appear to have clinically significant effects on bioavailable endogenous androgens. Many women whose menopause-related symptoms and bone loss responded inadequately to estrogen therapy were found to benefit from the addition of androgens.

Sarrel PM. Sexual dysfunction: treat or refer. Obstet Gynecol. 2005;106:834–9. Annotation: Sexual dysfunction is common in post-menopausal women and may be caused by several factors. Listening to the patient and clarifying her concerns are important. The nature of the problem needs to be defined, its severity and duration, and her motivation for treatment established. A complete physical evaluation, including a pelvic examination and measurement of post-menopausal hormone levels, may provide important information for structuring a treatment plan.

Somboonporn W. Testosterone therapy for postmenopausal women: efficacy and safety. Semin Reprod Med. 2006;24:115–24. Annotation: Evidence exists that the use of testosterone in combination with hormone therapy has both benefits and risks. The benefits are an improvement in sexual function and an improved sense of wellbeing. The use of testosterone may be justified in specific clinical circumstances and should be limited to short-term use; long-term studies are not available.

Utian WH, MacLean DB, Symonds T, Symons J, Somayaji V, Sisson M. A methodology study to validate a structured diagnostic method used to diagnose female sexual dysfunction and its subtypes in postmenopausal women. J Sex Marital Ther. 2005;31:271–83. Annotation: A structured diagnostic method was developed to diagnose sexual dysfunction in post-menopausal women. The results showed that the method had good reliability. The structured diagnostic method can reliably diagnose female sexual dysfunction status and subtypes in post-menopausal women.

Metabolic Syndrome

According to the American Heart Association and the National Heart, Lung, and Blood Institute, having three or more of the following: waist circumference equal to or greater than 35 inches; blood pressure equal to or greater than 130/85 mmHg; fasting glucose equal to or greater than 100 mg/dl; triglyceride blood tests (taken during cholesterol measurements) equal to or greater than 150 mg/dl; or HDL cholesterol (the "good" cholesterol) less than 50 mg/dl is consistent with the condition of metabolic syndrome. Metabolic syndrome has become increasingly common in women in the United States.

Having metabolic syndrome means having several disorders at the same time, all related to your metabolism. These disorders include: obesity, particularly excess fat tissue around the waist or abdomen (having an "apple shape"); elevated blood pressure; elevated level of triglycerides, the blood fat, and low level of high-density lipoprotein (HDL) cholesterol, the "good" cholesterol, fostering plaque buildup in artery walls; and resistance to insulin, the key hormone from the pancreas that helps regulate your blood sugar level, resulting in elevated blood sugar. In addition, in metabolic syndrome, there is increased inflammation of the lining cells of the blood vessels. This is characterized by high blood levels of chemical markers of inflammation, such as C-reactive protein. Finally, in metabolic syndrome, there is an increased tendency for blood clotting, as evidenced by high levels of fibrinogen or plasminogen activator inhibitor-1.

Women with metabolic syndrome are at increased risk for type 2 diabetes and coronary heart disease, as well as other diseases related to plaque buildup in artery walls, including stroke and peripheral vascular disease. There are new data that women with metabolic syndrome have not only high levels of C-reactive protein but less sexual function and less sexual satisfaction.

The primary goal of clinical management of the metabolic syndrome is to reduce the risk for cardiovascular disease and type 2 diabetes. This can be achieved with the following lifestyle interventions: weight loss to achieve a desirable weight; increased physical activity with a goal of at least 30 minutes of moderate-intensity activity on most days of the week; and healthy eating habits such as the Mediterranean diet. Medications may be needed to reduce LDL cholesterol, blood pressure, and glucose values to recommended levels. Women who smoke should stop smoking. Women with sexual health problems may need to be referred to a sexual medicine healthcare provider.

References for Metabolic Syndrome:

Esposito K, Pontillo A, Di Palo C, Giugliano G, Masella M, Marfella R, Giugliano D. Effect of weight loss and lifestyle changes on vascular inflammatory markers in obese women: a randomized trial. JAMA. 2003;289:1799–804. Annotation: A total of 120 pre-menopausal obese women aged 20–46 years without diabetes, hypertension or hyperlipidemia participated in a randomized, single-blind trial using a low-energy Mediterranean-style diet. After 2 years, body mass index decreased more in the intervention group than in controls, as did serum concentrations of interleuken-6, interleuken-18, and C-reactive protein. A multidisciplinary program aimed to reduce body weight in obese women through lifestyle changes was associated with a reduction in markers of vascular inflammation.

Esposito K, Marfella R, Ciotola M, Di Palo C, Giugliano F, Giugliano G, D'Armiento M, D'Andrea F, Giugliano D. Effect of a mediterranean-style diet on endothelial dysfunction and markers of vascular inflammation in the metabolic syndrome: a randomized trial. JAMA. 2004;292:1440–6. Annotation: A total of 180 patients (81 women) with the metabolic syndrome participated in a trial involving a Mediterranean-style diet of daily consumption of whole grains, fruits, vegetables, nuts, and olive oil. After 2 years, patients following the Mediterranean-style diet were observed to have significantly reduced serum concentrations of C-reactive protein, interleuken-6, interleuken-7, and interleuken-18, as well as decreased insulin resistance, compared to the control group.

Esposito K, Ciotola M, Marfella R, Di Tommaso D, Cobellis L, Giugliano D. Sexual dysfunction in women with the metabolic syndrome. Diabetes Care. 2005;28:756. Annotation: A total of 100 pre-menopausal women were enrolled if they had three or more of the criteria to meet the diagnosis of the metabolic syndrome. A total of 100 women without metabolic syndrome served as the control group. Compared with the control group, women with the metabolic syndrome had a reduced mean total Female Sexual Function Index score. A score was considered good >30/36; intermediate 23–29/36; and poor <23/36. A total of 77% of the control women had a Female Sexual Function Index score considered good, 21% had intermediate, and 2% had poor. Women with the metabolic syndrome had scores that were significantly lower at 55%, 36%, and 9%, respectively.

Esposito K, Ciotola M, Marfella R, Di Tommaso D, Cobellis L, Giugliano D. The metabolic syndrome: a cause of sexual dysfunction in women. Int J Impot Res. 2005;17:224–6. Annotation: A total of 200 women participated, 80 in the control group and 120 with the metabolic syndrome. Women with the metabolic syndrome had reduced mean Female Sexual Function Index scores, reduced satisfaction rates, and higher circulating levels of C-reactive protein.

Giugliano F, Esposito K, Di Palo C, Ciotola M, Giugliano G, Marfella R, D'Armiento M, Giugliano D. Erectile dysfunction associates with endothelial dysfunction and raised proinflammatory cytokine levels in obese men. J Endocrinol Invest. 2004;27:665–9. Annotation: A total of 80 obese men were divided into two groups according to the presence or absence of erectile dysfunction. Compared with non-obese, age-matched men, obese men had higher circulating concentrations of the proinflammatory cytokines interleukin-6, interleukin-8, and interleukin-18, as well as C-reactive protein. C-reactive protein levels were significantly higher in obese men with erectile dysfunction as compared with obese men without erectile dysfunction.

Miller EL, Mitchell A. Metabolic syndrome: screening, diagnosis, and management. J Midwifery Womens Health. 2006;51:141–51. Annotation: Metabolic syndrome is a cluster of health findings that increase the risk of cardiovascular events. The prevalence of metabolic syndrome is higher in women and is linked to female sexual dysfunction.

Oral Contraception

Information in this section concerning oral contraceptive pills applies to other delivery systems, including patch and vaginal ring contraception, since all of these delivery systems use ethinyl estradiol and synthetic progesterone.

Most women spend decades of their lives avoiding pregnancy. Oral contraceptives are a widely used form of reversible contraception. They have been used by approximately 80% of American women born since 1945. Over 100 million women worldwide have used the oral contraceptive pill.

The good news about oral contraceptives is that there are multiple benefits associated with their use. Besides being a highly effective contraceptive agent that is completely reversible in terms of fertility when discontinued, use of the oral contraceptive increases control of the menstrual cycle and decreases the days of menstrual bleeding, the volume of menstrual blood, and the intensity and frequency of menstrual cramps. In addition, use of the oral contraceptive decreases the risk of ovarian and uterine cancer, as well as the occurrence of benign ovarian cysts, endometriosis, and pelvic inflammatory disease. Furthermore, oral contraceptives are effective treatments for acne and facial hair growth or hirsutism.

These benefits associated with oral contraceptive use may also positively influence a woman's interest in sex. A medication that is safe and effective and decreases the fear of unwanted pregnancy, painful gynecologic conditions, social inhibition and embarrassment from acne and hirsutism, and menstrual bleeding, can increase sexual interest. This is especially true if the partner does not share contraceptive concerns.

Oral contraceptives are made up of a synthetic estradiol, ethinyl estradiol, and a synthetic progesterone. The action of these two agents is to reduce metabolic activity of the ovary and suppress ovulation, effectively preventing pregnancy. Ethinyl estradiol is a highly potent sex steroid that has approximately 600 times more affinity for the estradiol receptor than the bioidentical 17 beta estradiol. Use of ethinyl estradiol leads to diminished FSH and LH and reduced ovarian metabolic activity with decreased circulating levels of androgens and estrogens. Oral contraception causes a marked increase in hepatic synthesis of sex hormone binding globulin, the major binding protein for sex steroid hormones in the circulation. The result is a decrease in androgen hormone levels, in particular, unbound testosterone. Ethinyl estradiol-based contraception use is reported to be associated with sexual side effects. If oral contraceptives have a negative effect on women's sexual health, this negative sexual consequence could impact large numbers of women since so many women use the birth control pill.

The most commonly reported sexual side effects include diminished sexual interest, decreased frequency of sexual intercourse, diminished vaginal lubrication, decreased sexual arousal, and increased pain during intercourse. Several randomized, controlled trials have examined the effects of oral contraceptives on sexual function. While using a placebo control group allows for the determination of the independent effects of oral contraceptives on sexual health, this can prove difficult to achieve, as women must be safe from pregnancy, and therefore surgical sterilization of the woman or her partner is required for placebo control.

In 1978, Leeton and colleagues examined the sexual effects of oral contraceptives in women who had undergone surgical sterilization. In this trial, women who were established oral contraceptive users were randomized to either receive an oral contraceptive for one month and then placebo for the next month, or the same treatments in reverse order. During both months, participants answered questions related to sexual health and compared their current experiences with the previous month. There was significant reduction in sexual function during oral contraceptive compared to placebo use.

In 1993, Graham and colleagues examined the effects of oral contraceptives on sexuality as part of a trial to examine efficacy of oral contraceptives for the treatment of pre-menstrual syndrome. Participants were randomized to receive oral contraceptive or placebo. At baseline and over three months, participants were asked to rate their daily levels of sexual interest. The study results suggested decreased sexual interest was associated with oral contraceptive use.

In another investigation, Graham and colleagues performed a randomized, placebo-controlled clinical trial to examine the effects of oral contraceptive use on sexual function, publishing their results in 1995. Sterilized women or women with sterilized partners were randomized to receive either a combined oral contraceptive, a progesterone-only pill or a placebo for four months. Standardized, structured interviews and questionnaires were used to assess women's sexual function. Women subjects were from Scotland or the Philippines. At the end of the trial, among the Scottish women but not the Philippine women, ratings of sexual interest and sexual activity declined in the combined oral contraceptive group but not in the progesterone-only pill or placebo groups. The authors concluded that the reactions to oral contraceptives depended, in part, on baseline user characteristics. Negative changes in sexuality associated with oral contraceptive use were greater among women with a more positive experience of their sexuality at baseline (Scottish women) than among women with a more negative experience of their sexuality at baseline (Philippine women).

In 2006, Panzer and colleagues examined the effects of oral contraceptives on the blood level of sex hormone binding globulin. The control group consisted of women who had never used oral contraceptives, comparing them to women who had discontinued use of the birth control pill or continued to use it. Women who were never users had higher levels of sexual interest and lower levels of sexual pain during intercourse compared to continued users or discontinued users of oral contraceptives. An additional finding of their study was that total testosterone was a poor test to evaluate the androgen status in women who had ever used oral contraception. Assessments of "unbound" testosterone, such as calculated free testosterone, were more useful to assess androgen status in those women who had ever used an oral contraceptive. Finally, Panzer and colleagues found that the sex hormone binding globulin values in ever users were 400% higher than in never users. After discontinuation of oral contraceptives, sex hormone binding globulin levels remained almost twice as high as that of never users. They concluded that further research was needed to investigate the impact of oral contraceptives on androgen blood levels and women's sexual health issues.

There are other peer review publications concerning oral contraceptives and women's sexual health problems, in particular, increased sexual pain during intercourse. Berglund and colleagues examined over 150 Swedish women aged 12–26 years and found that 1/3 reported dyspareunia. Using oral contraception for more than 2 years was an independent variable increasing the risk of genital pain.

Bouchard and colleagues studied almost 140 women with vulvar vestibulitis whose symptoms had appeared in the previous 2 years and compared them to over 30 age-matched controls. A high risk of vulvar vestibulitis was found in the women who had ever used the oral contraceptive pill as compared to never users. The risk was even higher when oral contraceptive pills were first used before age 16, and the risk increased with duration of oral contraceptive pill use.

Bazin and colleagues examined almost 60 women, aged 18–35 years, with dyspareunia for 6 months secondary to vulvar vestibulitis syndrome and over 170 women of similar age without dyspareunia. Women who had used oral contraceptives before age 17 had a higher risk of having dyspareunia compared to women who had never used oral contraceptive pills.

Goldstein and colleagues used the epidemiologic study "Sex in Sweden" to analyze data in over 800 sexually active pre-menopausal women. They found a strong association between dyspareunia and oral contraceptive pill use. This was in sharp contrast to sexually active pre-menopausal women who used, at their last intercourse, condoms or intrauterine devices for contraception. There was no association between condom and intrauterine device use with increased dyspareunia.

In summary, sexual health problems occur in context. Many influences can ultimately determine whether use of any agent causes a sexual health concern. In some women, the negative hormone effects may be associated with sexual health problems. The most popular non-hormonal contraceptive is an intrauterine device with locally added low dose progesterone (e.g., Mirena™). For some women, however, the increased contraceptive security, in particular in a new relationship, improvement in acne or decreased risk of such conditions as benign ovarian cysts and endometriosis may override the hormonally driven negative effects on sexual function. The most important fact is that if you are experiencing sexual side effects and have ever used oral contraceptives, consider seeking consultation with a healthcare provider or sexual medicine specialist.

References for Oral Contraceptives:

Bancroft J, Sartorius N. The effects of oral contraceptives on well-being and sexuality. Oxf Rev Reprod Biol. 1990;12:57–92. Annotation: There are conflicting reports on improved and adverse effects of pills on sexuality and libido, implying that pill choice confounds the results, libido cycles are altered, or subtle effects of steroids on sexual response are overwhelmed by psychosocial factors in some women.

Coenen CM, Thomas CM, Borm GF, Hollanders JM, Rolland R. Changes in androgens during treatment with four low-dose contraceptives. Contraception. 1996;53:171–6. Annotation: One hundred women were randomized to receive 1 of 4 oral contraceptives over 6 months. Mean serum sex hormone binding globulin increased significantly in all 4 groups. There were significant decreases of serum testosterone. Oral contraceptive use changes the endogenous androgen environment in the direction of hypoandrogenism.

Davis AR, Castano PM. Oral contraceptives and libido in women. Annu Rev Sex Res. 2004;15:297–320. Annotation: Thirty original research studies were reviewed. In the 4 prospective and cross-sectional controlled studies, women using oral contraceptives reported both increased and decreased libido compared to non-oral contraceptive pill users. The findings from 5 randomized, placebo-controlled studies were mixed. In the most recent and well-conducted trial, a decrease in libido in oral contraceptive users compared to placebo users was found.

Graham CA, Sherwin BB. The relationship between mood and sexuality in women using an oral contraceptive as a treatment for premenstrual symptoms. Psychoneuroendocrinology. 1993;18:273–81. Annotation: A total of 45 women with pre-menstrual complaints were randomly assigned to receive either placebo or triphasic oral contraceptive for 3 months. Women who received the triphasic oral contraceptive reported decreased sexual interest during the menstrual and post-menstrual phases of the cycle. Oral contraceptives can directly influence women's sexuality.

Graham CA, Ramos R, Bancroft J, Maglaya C, Farley TM. The effects of steroidal contraceptives on the well-being and sexuality of women: a double-blind, placebo-controlled, two-centre study of combined and progestogen-only methods. Contraception. 1995;52:363–9. Annotation: A total of 150 women who had been sterilized or whose partners had been vasectomized were recruited from 2 locations, the Philippines and Scotland. Women were randomly assigned to 1 of 3 treatments: combined oral contraceptive, progestogen-only pill or placebo, and continued on treatment for 4 months. The combined oral contraceptive adversely affected sexuality in the Edinburgh women, with 12 of the 25 women in this group also reporting reduced sexual interest as a side effect.

Mango D, Ricci S, Manna P, Miggiano GA, Serra GB. Clinical and hormonal effects of ethinyl estradiol combined with gestodene and desogestrel in young women with acne vulgaris. Contraception. 1996;53:163–70. Annotation: Nineteen patients with post-pubertal acne vulgaris participated and were randomly allocated into 2 groups of different oral contraceptives. By the end of the third cycle of treatment, there was a 3-fold rise of the initial values of plasma sex hormone binding globulin. Both agents were good choices in the therapy of acne vulgaris.

Panzer C, Wise S, Fantini G, Kang D, Munarriz R, Guay A, Goldstein I. Impact of oral contraceptives on sex hormone-binding globulin and androgen levels: a retrospective study in women with sexual dysfunction. J Sex Med. 2006;3:104–13. Annotation: A total of 124 pre-menopausal women with sexual health complaints for >6 months participated. Sex hormone binding globulin values in the women who had been on oral contraceptives for >6 months and continued taking them were 4 times higher than those in the women who had never taken oral contraceptives. Despite a decrease in sex hormone binding globulin values after discontinuation of oral contraception, sex hormone binding globulin levels in women who had been on oral contraceptives for >6 months remained significantly elevated, in comparison with women who had never taken oral contraceptives. Long-term sexual, metabolic, and mental health consequences might result as a consequence of chronic sex hormone binding globulin elevation.

Sanders SA, Graham CA, Bass JL, Bancroft J. A prospective study of the effects of oral contraceptives on sexuality and well-being and their relationship to discontinuation. Contraception 2001;64:51–8. Annotation: Among the 79 women who participated, 47% discontinued oral contraceptives and 14% switched to a different oral contraceptive. Emotional side effects included worsening of premenstrual syndrome, decreased frequency of sexual thoughts, and decreased sexual arousal. Emotional and sexual side effects were the best predictors of discontinuation/switching.

Schaffir J. Hormonal contraception and sexual desire: a critical review. J Sex Marital Ther. 2006;32:305–14. Annotation: Effects on sexual desire most likely represent a complex combination of biological, psychological, and social effects.

Sobbrio GA, Granata A, D'Arrigo F, Arena D, Panacea A, Trimarchi F, Granese D, Pulle C. Treatment of hirsutism related to micropolycystic ovary syndrome (MPCO) with two low-dose oestrogen oral contraceptives: a comparative randomized evaluation. Acta Eur Fertil. 1990;21:139–41. Annotation: A total of 34 young women with excessive body hair participated and were randomly assigned to 1 of 2 oral contraceptive pill groups. A significant decrease in total testosterone and free testosterone was observed. Sex hormone binding globulin increased significantly.

Sobbrio GA, Granata A, Granese D, D'Arrigo F, Panacea A, Nicita R, Pulle C, Trimarchi F. Sex hormone binding globulin, cortisol binding globulin, thyroxine binding globulin, ceruloplasmin: changes in treatment with two oral contraceptives low in oestrogen. Clin Exp Obstet Gynecol. 1991;18:43–5. Annotation: Forty young, normally cycling healthy volunteers were randomly assigned to 2 different oral contraceptives. A marked significant increase in all the carrier proteins was found, especially sex hormone binding globulin. The increase in sex hormone binding globulin, cortisol binding globulin, thyroxine binding globulin, and seruloplasmin is an expression of the estrogenicity of the oral contraceptives studied.

Persistent Genital Arousal Disorder

Persistent genital arousal disorder (PGAD), also known as persistent sexual arousal syndrome (PSAS), is an uncommon sexual dysfunction that can significantly interfere with a woman's quality of life. The spontaneous, intrusive, and unwanted genital arousal and sexual tension (e.g., tingling, throbbing, pulsating) symptoms are persistent and recurrent, leaving some victims feeling humiliated, confused, isolated, frustrated, self-conscious, and shamed. There are no known and recognized safe and effective treatments that cure persistent genital arousal disorder. The symptoms can become so severe and unrelenting that some women become suicidal.

An evolving neurologic/biologic-based hypothesis is that persistent genital arousal disorder is related to a group of "uninhibited neurons" within the central anatomical structures or networks involved in the regulation of women's genital arousal. These "uninhibited neurons" lack appropriate inhibition/excitation neurotransmitter regulation and, as a result, the balance is shifted toward excitation, consistent with recurrent "focal seizure" activity.

Current strategies for persistent genital arousal disorder aim to maximize "PGAD-free time" and include engaging in: repeated intense orgasms; mental and physical distractions and refusal to give in to the horrible sensations; hypnosis; methodologies to diminish perineal sensation; and administration of selective serotonin reuptake inhibitors or anti-seizure medications.

References for Persistent Genital Arousal Disorder:

Amsterdam A, Abu-Rustum N, Carter J, Krychman M. Persistent sexual arousal syndrome associated with increased soy intake. J Sex Med. 2005;2:338–40. Annotation: This is a case study of a 44-year-old woman who reported 5–6 months of increased pelvic tension not associated with an increase in desire requiring her to self-stimulate to orgasm approximately 15 times daily. Upon further inquiry, the patient disclosed that her dietary regimen included soy intake in excess of 4 pounds per day that began approximately 1 month prior to the onset of symptoms. Treatment consisted of supportive counseling and dietary modification. At the 3-month follow-up visit, the patient's sexual complaints resolved.

Freed L. Persistent sexual arousal syndrome. J Sex Med. 2005;2:743. Annotation: Abrupt discontinuation of selective serotonin reuptake inhibitors anti-depressants may be the cause of persistent genital arousal disorder.

Goldmeier D, Bell C, Richardson D. Withdrawal of selective serotonin reuptake inhibitors (SSRIs) may cause increased atrial natriuretic peptide (ANP) and persistent sexual arousal in women? J Sex Med. 2006;3:376. Annotation: Abrupt discontinuation of selective serotonin reuptake inhibitors may be the cause of persistent genital arousal disorder. The mechanism may be via changed neurotransmitters.

Goldmeier D, Leiblum SR. Persistent genital arousal in women—a new syndrome entity. Int J STD AIDS. 2006;17:215–6. Annotation: Women with persistent genital arousal disorder become involuntarily aroused genitally for extended periods of time in the absence of sexual desire. These women are usually found to be very distressed. A number of women report symptoms after withdrawal from selective serotonin reuptake inhibitors.

Leiblum SR, Nathan SG. Persistent sexual arousal syndrome: a newly discovered pattern of female sexuality. J Sex Marital Ther. 2001;27:365–80. Annotation: Persistent genital arousal disorder has not been noted or described in the previous sexuality, psychiatric or medical literature. The woman's complaint is of excessive and often unremitting arousal. There is persistent physiological arousal in the absence of conscious feelings of sexual desire.

Leiblum S, Brown C, Wan J, Rawlinson L. Persistent sexual arousal syndrome: a descriptive study. J Sex Med. 2005;2:331–7. Annotation: A total of 103 respondents participated in a 46-item Internet survey. Involuntary genital and clitoral arousal persisting for extended time periods, genital arousal unrelated to subjective feelings of sexual desire, and genital arousal not relieved with orgasms were the most frequently endorsed features associated with this syndrome. Symptom triggers included sexual stimulation, masturbation, stress, and anxiety. Distress about the condition was high in 40% of respondents. The strongest predictors of distress were intrusive and unwanted feelings of genital arousal, continuous symptoms, feelings of unhappiness, shame and worry, and reduced sexual satisfaction.

Low NN, Low RB. Persistent sexual arousal syndrome—a descriptive study. J Sex Med. 2005;2:744. Annotation: Women with persistent genital arousal disorder, sufficiently disturbed by the condition to seek medical help, can report severe distraction, generally high levels of distress, and sometimes-suicidal ideation. Internet surveys, as opposed to doctor visits, are problematic. Such surveys include a proportion of their sample population as feeling: pleased (29%), youthful (21%), happy (20%), and glad (18%), suggesting that these survey respondents are reporting something else.

Wylie K, Levin R, Hallam-Jones R, Goddard A. Sleep exacerbation of persistent sexual arousal syndrome in a postmenopausal woman. J Sex Med. 2006;3:296–302. Annotation: In one post-menopausal woman, persistent genital arousal disorder was exacerbated by sleep onset. On becoming drowsy and falling lightly asleep in the laboratory, the vaginal blood flow increased by 95% of the basal value, confirming the subject's complaint of persistent sexual arousal during sleep. There was no evidence of malfunction of the brain, spinal cord, or pelvic area by MRI, but genito-sensory analysis of the clitoral and vaginal area showed evidence of reduced sensory function. Risperidone has been effective allowing the subject to sleep throughout the night without disturbance.

Yero AS, McKinney T, Petrides G, Goldstein I, Kellner CH, Successful Use of Electroconvulsive Therapy in 2 Cases of Persistent Sexual Arousal Syndrome and Bipolar Disorder, J ECT. 2006;22:274-5. Annotation: These are the first published cases documenting the successful use of electroconvulsive therapy in women with persistent genital arousal disorder.

Thyroid Conditions

Hormones are critical for sexual function. Like the sex hormones estrogen, testosterone, and progesterone, thyroid hormones act on cells to direct the synthesis and release of various proteins. Most cells in the body depend upon thyroid hormone for regulation of cellular metabolism. For example, thyroid hormone acts on the smooth muscle cells of the erectile tissues of the genitalia, including the clitoris, labia, and vagina, to increase cellular activity.

The thyroid gland is prone to several distinct problems. Too little production of thyroid hormone is called hypothyroidism; too much production is called hyperthyroidism. Hypothyroidism is much more common than hyperthyroidism.

It is estimated that as many as 10% of American women have some degree of thyroid hormone deficiency. Millions of women with sexual health problems don't realize they may have thyroid problems. Hypothyroid symptoms are non-specific and may include fatigue and weakness; weight gain or increased difficulty losing weight; coarse, dry hair and dry, rough, pale skin; hair loss; intolerance to cold; muscle cramps and frequent muscle aches; constipation; depression; irritability; memory loss; abnormal menstrual cycles; and sexual dysfunction. You may have any number of these symptoms, only one symptom or none at all. In some cases, symptoms may be so subtle or have been accepted for so long as being normal they are essentially not recognized.

There are different causes of hyperthyroidism, however, symptoms are usually the same regardless of the cause. Typically the onset of hyperthyroidism is very gradual, so women with the condition don't even realize they are experiencing symptoms. The increase in body metabolism can cause women with hyperthyroidism to experience: feeling hotter than those around them; losing weight even when eating more; fatigue at the end of the day and trouble sleeping; trembling hands; a hard or irregular heartbeat or palpitations; and irritability and a tendency to become easily upset. The weight issue may be confusing since some women experience an increase in appetite that does result in weight gain.

What are the sexual consequences of hypothyroidism and hyperthyroidism? Unfortunately, there are limited studies examining the sexual health of women with thyroid conditions. Salonia and colleagues examined the sexual function of 30 women with hypothyroidism and 18 women with hyperthyroidism, comparing the data to a control group of healthy age-matched women. As a group, those women with thyroid disorders had significantly worse lubrication and orgasm and significantly more sexual pain compared with the control group. Obviously, more research is needed in this area.

In summary, when a woman has a sexual health problem, assessment of thyroid function, along with other biologic determinations and other potential concomitant psychologic and interpersonal concerns should be addressed.

References for Thyroid Conditions:

Carani C, Isidori AM, Granata A, Carosa E, Maggi M, Lenzi A, Jannini EA. Multicenter study on the prevalence of sexual symptoms in male hypo- and hyperthyroid patients. J Clin Endocrinol Metab. 2005;90:6472–9. Annotation: Many patients with thyroid hormone disorders experience some sexual dysfunctions, which can be reversed by normalizing thyroid hormone levels.

Kilicarslan H, Bagcivan I, Yildirim MK, Sarac B, Kaya T. Effect of hypothyroidism on the NO/cGMP pathway of corpus cavernosum in rabbits. J Sex Med. 2006;3:830–7. Annotation: Erectile tissue in hypothyroid rabbits showed abnormalities compared with controls. Hypothyroidism may result in a decreased release of nitric oxide from nerves and from the blood vessel lining. Hypothyroidism may result in changes to neurotransmitter receptor density.

Veronelli A, Masu A, Ranieri R, Rognoni C, Laneri M, Pontiroli AE. Prevalence of erectile dysfunction in thyroid disorders: comparison with control subjects and with obese and diabetic patients. Int J Impot Res. 2006;18:111–4. Annotation: Erectile dysfunction was more frequent in patients affected by thyroid diseases (59%) than in controls (30%). The erectile dysfunction score was worse in thyroid patients than in control subjects.

Weber G, Vigone MC, Stroppa L, Chiumello G. Thyroid function and puberty. J Pediatr Endocrinol Metab. 2003;16:S253–7. Annotation: Thyroid hormones are essential for normal growth and sexual development. During puberty, changes in thyroid functions and an increase in thyroid volume occur as an adaptation to sexual development. Hypothyroidism diagnosed late in pre-pubertal years can cause a delay of puberty.

Vulvodynia

Vulvodynia is a chronic pain disorder localized to the vulvar region, lasting at least 3–6 months, with various clinical presentations. Associated with varying pain intensities and triggers, vulvodynia pain may be unremitting, intermittent or episodic; more intense at a certain time in the menstrual cycle or occurring only with touch. Symptoms of vulvar burning and itching may also vary. Pain in the vulvar region causes bother and concern and can have significant negative consequences on interpersonal and psychological wellbeing.

Various studies have shown that vulvodynia affects approximately 15% to 20% of adult women. In vulvodynia patients when compared to women without vulvodynia, studies have shown vulvar tissues to have more redness. Biopsies have shown more areas of chronic inflammation and more pain nerve fibers in vulvodynia patients as well. On physical examination of the pelvic floor, women with vulvodynia have increased spasm and increased tone of the levator ani muscle in response to vulvar pain. Unfortunately, despite vulvodynia being relatively common and often associated with high distress, there are minimal evidence-based data to guide health care professionals in the management of women with vulvodynia.

The underlying cause of vulvodynia is uncertain. It is possible that vulvodynia may actually be the result of many different causes. These may include inflammatory and infectious disease processes, neurologic conditions, genetic factors, stress factors, and hormone factors. As a result, one management strategy for all women with complaints of vulvar pain will likely not be successful.

If the vulvar pain is localized more to the region of the vestibule, it is a subtype of vulvodynia, commonly called vestibulitis or vulvar vestibulitis syndrome or vestibular adenitis. The cause of vulvar vestibulitis syndrome is also not known.

If the cause of the chronic vulvar pain is known, medical attention can then be directed to the underlying cause. Some examples of known causes of vulvar pain include: vulvovaginal Candida or yeast infections, endometriosis of the vulva, lichen sclerosis or lichen plannus of the vulva, contact dermatitis of the vulva, atrophy of the vulva from low levels of sex steroid hormones, pudendal nerve entrapment syndrome, referred pain from tender pelvic floor muscles, post-operative painful vulva after perineal surgery, painful vulva following pelvic or perineal radiation therapy for cancer, and other pain syndromes including referred pain misdiagnosed as coming from the vulva. Pain in the perineum can actually come from the urethra such as from urethritis, from the bladder such as from interstitial cystitis or even from the coccyx area. Risk factors for the development of vulvar pain include irritable bowel syndrome, interstitial cystitis, and oral contraceptive pills.

One of the most distressing aspects of vulvodynia is that afflicted women frequently experience pain for many months, often years, before being diagnosed. Many women with chronic vulvar pain are told that their symptoms are "all in their head," implying that their pain is not real. Lack of a diagnosis may further increase the distress caused by the vulvodynia and delay access to more specialized medical care often needed for this condition.

When the cause of chronic vulvar pain is not known or is at best uncertain, treatment interventions vary. Many health care professionals combine treatments including psychotherapy and/or behavioral counseling, pain medication, pelvic floor physical therapy, hormone treatments if indicated, and, as a last treatment option, surgical removal of portions of the affected vestibule. More research is needed to better understand how to manage vulvodynia.

References for Vulvodynia:

Bachmann GA, Rosen R, Pinn VW, Utian WH, Ayers C, Basson R, Binik YM, Brown C, Foster DC, Gibbons JM Jr, Goldstein I, Graziottin A, Haefner HK, Harlow BL, Spadt SK, Leiblum SR, Masheb RM, Reed BD, Sobel JD, Veasley C, Wesselmann U, Witkin SS. Vulvodynia: a state-of-the-art consensus on definitions, diagnosis and management. J Reprod Med. 2006;51:447–56. Annotation: Vulvodynia is a chronic pain syndrome affecting approximately 1 in 5 women. The causes, diagnosis, and treatment have not been clearly delineated.

Bergeron S, Binik YM, Khalife S, Pagidas K, Glazer HI, Meana M, Amsel R. A randomized comparison of group cognitive-behavioral therapy, surface electromyographic biofeedback, and vestibulectomy in the treatment of dyspareunia resulting from vulvar vestibulitis. Pain. 2001;91:297–306. Annotation: This study of 78 women compared 12-week trials of group cognitive-behavioral therapy and surface electromyographic biofeedback and surgery (vestibulectomy) in the treatment of dyspareunia resulting from vulvar vestibulitis. As compared with pre-treatment, study completers of all treatment groups reported statistically significant reductions on pain measures at post-treatment and 6-month follow-up, although the surgery (vestibulectomy) group was significantly more successful than the two other groups.

Brauer M, Laan E, ter Kuile MM. Sexual arousal in women with superficial dyspareunia. Arch Sex Behav. 2006;35:191–200. Annotation: Fifty women with dyspareunia and 25 women without sexual problems were studied. Women with dyspareunia had comparable levels of genital arousal to 2 different visual sexual stimuli as women without sexual complaints. With adequate visual sexual stimulation, women with dyspareunia showed equal levels of genital sexual arousal to visual sexual stimuli as women without sexual complaints, therefore, there was no evidence for impaired genital responsiveness associated with dyspareunia.

Goldstein AT, Klingman D, Christopher K, Johnson C, Marinoff SC. Surgical treatment of vulvar vestibulitis syndrome: outcome assessment derived from a postoperative questionnaire. J Sex Med. 2006;3:923–31. Annotation: A total of 134 women with vulvar vestibulitis syndrome underwent complete vulvar vestibulectomy with vaginal advancement surgery in a 5-year period. Of the 104 women interviewed in follow-up, 97 women were satisfied or very satisfied with the outcome of their surgery. Only 3 patients reported persistently worse symptoms after surgery, and only 7 reported permanent recurrence of any symptoms after surgery. Prior to surgery, 72% of the women were unable to have intercourse; however, after surgery, only 11% were unable to have intercourse.

Gordon AS. Clitoral pain: the great unexplored pain in women. J Sex Marital Ther. 2002;28:S123–8. Annotation: Clitoral pain is not often reported by patients or in literature. The author reports on 21 women who had clitoral pain as a major symptom. Features included mild to moderate rest pain and significant contact, light-touch induced or pressure induced pain. Associations include Multiple Sclerosis, Guillain Barre Syndrome, urethral sphincter dyssynergia, various vulvar pain syndromes (9 cases), post-hysterectomy, Lichen Sclerosis (5 cases), spondylolisthesis, vaginismus, and genital or pelvic trauma.

Graziottin A. Etiology and diagnosis of coital pain. J Endocrinol Invest. 2003;26: S115–21. Annotation: Coital pain is the leading symptom of 2 major sexual disorders, dyspareunia and vaginismus. Biological factors include hormonal, inflammatory, muscular, iatrogenic, neurologic, vascular, connective, and immunitary causes. Psychosexual factors—loss of libido and arousal disorders, associated with, or secondary to, sexual pain related disorders—may contribute to the worsening of coital pain over time, alone or when associated with couple problems. The clinical approach should aim at diagnosing biological, psychosexual, and context-dependent etiologies.

Masheb RM, Lozano-Blanco C, Kohorn EI, Minkin MJ, Kerns RD. Assessing sexual function and dyspareunia with the Female Sexual Function Index (FSFI) in women with vulvodynia. J Sex Marital Ther. 2004;30:315–24. Annotation: A total of 42 women with vulvodynia were assessed. Women with vulvodynia reported significantly worse overall sexual function than women without sexual dysfunction and greater pain with sexual intercourse than women with female sexual arousal disorder.

McElhiney J, Kelly S, Rosen R, Bachmann G. Satyriasis: the antiquity term for vulvodynia? J Sex Med. 2006;3:161–3. Annotation: Vulvodynia is a condition reported to affect approximately 15% to 27% of women. Vulvodynia was not discussed or reported in traditional medical textbooks until the end of the 1800's. The authors proposed that vulvodynia was described as far back as the 1st century CE by Soranus as "satyriasis in females."

Reissing ED, Brown C, Lord MJ, Binik YM, Khalife S. Pelvic floor muscle functioning in women with vulvar vestibulitis syndrome. J Psychosom Obstet Gynaecol. 2005;26:107–13. Annotation: A total of 29 women with vulvar vestibulitis syndrome were matched to 29 women with no pain with intercourse. Women with vulvar vestibulitis syndrome demonstrated significantly more vaginal hypertonicity, lack of vaginal muscle strength, and restriction of the vaginal opening, compared to women with no pain with intercourse. Pelvic floor pathology in women with vulvar vestibulitis syndrome is reactive in nature and elicited with palpations that result in vulvar vestibulitis syndrome-type pain. Treatment interventions need to recognize the critical importance of addressing the conditioned, protective muscle guarding response in women with vulvar vestibulitis syndrome.

Sadownik LA. Clinical profile of vulvodynia patients. A prospective study of 300 patients. J Reprod Med. 2000;45:679–84. Annotation: A total of 301 patients with vulvodynia, average age was 38 years, completed a questionnaire. Patients reported dyspareunia (71%), vulvar burning (57%), and vulvar itching (46%). One-third reported problems with sexual response. Over 64% of the time, all therapeutic interventions tried by patients made the vulvar symptoms no better or worse.

ter Kuile MM, Weijenborg PT. A cognitive-behavioral group program for women with vulvar vestibulitis syndrome (VVS): factors associated with treatment success. J Sex Marital Ther. 2006;32:199–213. Annotation: This study in 76 women with vulvar vestibulitis syndrome indicates that a cognitive-behavioral group program affects sexuality, pain control, vaginal muscle control, and vestibular pain. These changes may mediate alterations in pain during intercourse. Improvements in sexual functioning and vestibular pain during treatment seem to be particularly important factors in determining short and longer term treatment outcome.

Weijmar Schultz WC, Gianotten WL, van der Meijden WI, van de Wiel HB, Blindeman L, Chadha S, Drogendijk AC. Behavioral approach with or without surgical intervention to the vulvar vestibulitis syndrome: a prospective randomized and non-randomized study. J Psychosom Obstet Gynaecol. 1996;17:143–8. Annotation: The behavioral approach should be the first choice of treatment for vulvar vestibulitis syndrome. Surgical intervention should be considered as an additional form of treatment in some cases of vulvar vestibulitis syndrome to facilitate breaking the vicious circle of irritation, pelvic floor muscle hypertonia, and sexual maladaptive behavior.

Weijmar Schultz W, Basson R, Binik Y, Eschenbach D, Wesselmann U, Van Lankveld J. Women's sexual pain and its management. J Sex Med. 2005;2:301–16. Annotation: There is increasing evidence for the role of neuropathic pain mechanisms in the pathophysiology of sexual pain disorders. Studies reveal that differentiation between vaginismus and dyspareunia using clinical tools is difficult. The traditional treatment of vaginismus with vaginal "dilatation" plus psycho-education, desensitization, etc. is not evidence-based; the pelvic floor musculature is indirectly innervated by the limbic system and highly reactive to emotional stimuli and states. Pelvic floor therapies for dyspareunia may be effective but long-term studies are needed.

Wylie K, Hallam-Jones R, Harrington C. Psychological difficulties within a group of patients with vulvodynia. J Psychosom Obstet Gynaecol. 2004;25:257–65. Annotation: A total of 164 women (82 with vulvodynia and 82 in a control group) were studied. The level of psychological difficulties revealed significantly higher levels of psychological distress in the vulvodynia group within the domains of somatisation, obsessive-compulsive behavior, depression, anxiety, and phobic symptoms, as well as with interpersonal sensitivity hostility and paranoia.

Effects Of Psychologic Factors on Female Sexual Function

Sandra Leiblum, Ph.D.

Director, Center for Sexual and Relationship Health
Robert Wood Johnson Medical School
Piscataway, New Jersey

Psychologic Factors

Although ideally women would enjoy problem-free, easily arousing, gratifying sex, far too many women complain of an array of sexual inhibitions, from concerns about being seen naked to worries about their smells, sounds or sensations during sex. There are usually a variety of factors at play here. Typically, a host of past and present contributions, or what we sometimes think of as predisposing, precipitating, maintaining, and contextual factors, are responsible for sexual discontents and difficulties.

Predisposing factors that may set the stage for later sexual problems include: constitutional (e.g., illness, anatomical deformities) and early life experiences, such as negative, neglectful or critical parents; an upbringing that invests sex with negative messages about sex or men; untrustworthy or disappointing relationships; or past experiences of sexual, physical or emotional abuse or violence.

Precipitating factors are the immediate triggers for sexual problems. Although they vary enormously, they may include such experiences as an unwanted or traumatic first sexual experience, repeated criticisms from a spouse, the discovery of a partner's infidelity or even a single episode of sexual humiliation. Repetitive or traumatic sexual experiences challenge or damage self-confidence and may be pathonomic for sexual dysfunction, even in reasonably resilient individuals.

Finally, maintaining factors such as relationship distress, performance anxiety, guilt, inadequate sexual information or stimulation, psychiatric disorders (especially high anxiety and depression), loss of attraction for a partner, impaired self-image or self-esteem, restricted foreplay, poor communication, and lack of privacy may prolong and exacerbate problems, irrespective of the original predisposing or precipitating conditions. Maintaining factors also include contextual factors that can interfere or interrupt sexual activity, such as environmental constraints or anger/resentment towards a partner.

Should predisposing or precipitating psychologic factors cause you distress, please consider consulting the sexual medicine healthcare professional.

References:

Althof SE, Leiblum SR, Chevert-Measson M, Hartman U, Levine SB, McCabe M, Plaut M, Rodrigues O, Wylie K. Psychological and Interpersonal Contributions to Male and Female Sexual Function and Dysfunction. In TF Lue, R Basson, R Rosen, F Giuliano, S Khoury, F Montorsi (eds), Sexual Dysfunctions in Men and Women (2004) Health Publications, Paris, pp. 73-116. Annotation: A comprehensive, evidence-based review of the most salient psychological and relational contributions to predisposing, precipitating, and maintaining sexual dysfunction in men and women.

Leiblum S, Wiegel M. Psychotherapeutic interventions for treating female sexual dysfunction. World J Urol. 2002;20:127–136. Annotation: A review of cognitive behavioral treatments for women's sexual dysfunctions, with a description of each of the various interventions.

Titta M, Tavolini IM, Moro FD, Cisternino A, Bassi P. Sexual counseling improved erectile rehabilitation after non-nerve-sparing radical retropubic prostatectomy or cystectomy—results of a randomized prospective study. J Sex Med. 2006;3:267–73. Annotation: In this prospective randomized study, patients were divided into two groups: 29 patients were treated with sexual counseling and intracavernosal therapy; 28 were treated with only intracavernosal therapy. At the end of the study, for those patients who received sexual counseling, there were significantly higher total International Index of Erectile Function scores, higher scores of sexual satisfaction, sexual desire, orgasmic function, and general satisfaction, significantly more patients became responders to home sildenafil, and there were significantly fewer dropout cases.

Medical Therapies for Female Sexual Dysfunction

Irwin Goldstein, M.D.

Director, Sexual Medicine
Alvarado Hospital, San Diego, California
Editor-in-Chief, The Journal of Sexual Medicine

Androgen Therapy

Androgens and androgen precursors consist of 7 different 19-carbon sex steroids. Androgens are naturally synthesized from cholesterol by the ovary and the adrenal gland. They are also synthesized from androgen precursors in multiple peripheral organs, such as the skeletal muscle and skin. These androgen and androgen precursor hormones are likely important for tissue structure and function; 4 of the 7 may be clinically measured: dehydroepiandrosterone, androstenedione, testosterone, and dihydrotestosterone.

Androgen synthesis in your body is an example of a one-direction cascade or waterfall. Dehydroepiandrosterone, the first or precursor androgen, is converted by an enzyme into androstenedione, which is then converted by a different enzyme into testosterone, which is then converted by a different enzyme to dihydrotestosterone. This is clinically important information. Women with low dehydroepiandrosterone blood levels who consider dehydroepiandrosterone treatment can raise that level and the rest of the androgen levels from this conversion. In contrast, women with low testosterone blood levels who consider testosterone therapy raise only the testosterone and dihydrotestosterone levels. In androgen synthesis, you can't convert "backwards" into the early part of the synthetic cascade; you can only convert "forward" into the remaining portion.

It should be noted that both dehydroepiandrosterone and testosterone use can raise estradiol values in women. This action is due to testosterone converting to estradiol by the enzyme aromatase. This is likely why some women with hot flashes and night sweats report improvement in symptoms following systemic androgen or androgen precursor use without the need for or risk associated with systemic estrogen administration.

Androgens and androgen precursors have a profound effect on many physiological functions in women including: stimulation of sexual desire, interest, thoughts, and fantasies; regulation of genital (vaginal and clitoral) blood flow; amount and quality of vaginal lubrication; structural and functional integrity of the clitoris, prepuce, vaginal muscularis (smooth muscle layer), G-spot, and minor vestibular glands; stimulation of bone growth; increase in muscle mass; maintenance of energy and well-being; maintenance of lean body composition; control of oil gland activity in skin; and regulation of body hair growth.

Current evidence shows that androgens and androgen precursors achieve their multiple functions by entering body cells and copying or transcribing specific genetic information from the cell's nucleus onto biochemical messages that ultimately result in the synthesis of critical proteins. These critical proteins help maintain the structure and function of many genital (clitoris, vaginal muscularis, labia minora, G-spot, minor vestibular glands) and non-genital (brain, bone, skeletal muscle, skin) tissues.

Testosterone, a well-studied androgen, is an important hormone to continually direct and maintain various tissues in a healthy structure and function. Testosterone appears to be a vital component of women's sexual health and is an important factor in women's overall health, however women with low testosterone can still have a satisfactory sex life.

Before puberty, when all the androgens are low, the woman's peripheral genitals including the clitoris, prepuce (foreskin), frenulum, labia minora, labia majora, G-spot, and vestibule are not fully developed. After puberty, when androgen levels increase, the woman's peripheral genitals fully develop. The clitoris reaches adult size, sensitivity, and engorgement capability, the labia minora develop tissue mass and local lubrication occurs via a series of glands that release the lubricant onto the labia during sexual arousal. The vagina muscularis easily relaxes during sexual arousal so that the vagina increases appropriately in length and width. With aging or certain medications (e.g., oral contraceptives, infertility drugs, selective serotonin reuptake inhibitors), when androgen levels fall, the woman's androgen-dependent peripheral genitals, such as the clitoris and prepuce, undergo atrophy and take on the same underdeveloped characteristics they had prior to puberty. The message here is that the hormone testosterone is required throughout post-pubertal life to maintain genital tissue structure and function. This applies, as well, to the estrogen sex steroids.

Androgens are synthesized in multiple locations in the body. For many women, this means that even after menopause the body is still capable of synthesizing adequate amounts of androgens. Studies have shown that 90% of the androgen precursor dehydroepiandrosterone is synthesized in the adrenal gland, with the remaining 10% in the ovaries; the androgen precursor androstenedione is synthesized equally in the adrenal gland and ovary (40% in each) and 20% in the peripheral organs; whereas testosterone is synthesized 50% by the peripheral organs and 25% each in the adrenal gland and ovaries. Why is this clinically important information? The ovaries are, surprising to most individuals, critical organs not only for estrogen but also for androgen synthesis. Women thinking of having their ovaries removed as part of a hysterectomy procedure need to be aware that the ovaries do synthesize many critical androgens; if the ovaries are removed, remaining androgen sources may not be adequate to maintain genital tissue structure and function.

Women's androgen levels decline with age, beginning at age 30, and progress steadily downward. At 40, a woman's androgens are already half of the values they were at age 20. At 60, the androgen values are 1/3 of the values at age 20. Since these research studies are concerned with average values in large population samples, this does not mean that all women will have low testosterone. These studies do not report individual androgen blood test values.

Beyond aging, there are many other conditions or situations recognized to be associated with lower testosterone blood levels. The most common reason, however, is an elevation in the level of sex hormone binding globulin. Sex hormone binding globulin is produced by the liver cells and released into the blood stream. The purpose of sex hormone binding globulin is to bind the sex steroids (androgens, estrogens, and progestins) in the circulation. Androgens such as testosterone have a very high propensity or affinity to bind onto sex hormone binding globulin. What is important to understand is that for sex steroids in general, and testosterone in particular, it is the "unbound" form of hormone and not the hormone bound to sex hormone binding globulin that is the physiologically active form. In theory, it is the "unbound" form of testosterone that gets into the cell and directs the synthesis of important proteins. Therefore, the measurement of sex hormone binding globulin is of paramount importance in assessing the level of "unbound" testosterone in a woman with sexual health problems. In a woman, high sex hormone binding globulin levels pose a clinical problem. Sex hormone binding globulin values are increased by use of any estrogen (e.g., for contraception or treatment of menopausal symptoms), use of tamoxifen (for treatment of breast cancer), pregnancy, liver diseases (such as cirrhosis) or anti-seizure medications. Sex hormone binding globulin is lowered by androgen administration, a good bonus of testosterone use.

Low androgen blood test values may be caused by conditions that affect the ovaries. These include natural, surgical or premature menopause, injury to the ovaries by chemotherapy or radiation treatments for cancer, or systemic hormone treatments that affect the ovaries such as oral, patch or ring contraceptives, infertility hormone treatments, endometriosis hormone treatments or uterine fibroid hormone treatments.

If you fit the clinical symptoms of the syndrome called "androgen insufficiency" and have personal distress or bother, you may wish to consider treatment for low androgens. According to an international panel of experts, a syndrome of androgen insufficiency exists if the woman has any of the following symptoms: a diminished sense of well-being; feelings of helplessness or unhappiness; persistent or unexplained fatigue; sexual function changes such as decreased sexual interest, sexual receptivity, sexual pleasure, and/or decreased lubrication; or bone loss, decreased muscle strength, and/or changes of memory; in conjunction with having a blood test consistent with low "unbound" testosterone values.

Since there is no consensus as to what blood tests should be obtained when being evaluated for androgen insufficiency, the following list represents the personal opinion of the author of this section. Women should consider initially requesting the following androgen blood tests: dehydroepiandrosterone-sulfate: the sulfated form of dehydroepiandrosterone, more stable than dehydroepiandrosterone; total testosterone: values include both "bound" and "unbound" forms of testosterone; and sex hormone binding globulin: values enable the calculated free testosterone to be determined. Optional androgen blood tests include androstenedione and dihydrotestosterone.

There is a blood test called "free testosterone" (sometimes called "analog free testosterone") that theoretically measures only the "unbound" (and the most biologically important) form of testosterone. Unfortunately, this is currently not very accurate for technical reasons related to the specificity of the antibodies used. Relying on this test exclusively for diagnosis of androgen insufficiency may be misleading. While there are other accurate tests of "unbound testosterone," such as free androgen index and bioavailable testosterone, one recommended strategy is to use the free testosterone calculator available on the Internet. The value thus obtained is called the "calculated free testosterone." The "calculated free testosterone" is reliable and an easily available measure of "unbound" testosterone.

While these androgen blood tests are important, it is rare that the healthcare provider is only interested in the androgen status of a woman with sexual health concerns. Additional sex steroid hormone blood tests that are usually obtained include the following: estradiol: the most important estrogen, more meaningful in women in the transition or post-menopause; progesterone: the least understood as it relates to sexual medicine, although it appears to be involved in sexual interest and overall mood; follicle stimulating hormone and luteinizing hormone: measurements of the integrity of the pituitary gland and its role in monitoring estradiol values in a woman; prolactin: a potent inhibitor of sexual activity in a woman; and thyroid stimulating hormone: measurement of the integrity of the thyroid gland.

The results of these multiple tests need to be examined very carefully. Usually a pattern will emerge that helps the sexual medicine healthcare professional recommend a course of action. There is a clinically important controversy—the normal ranges of these blood tests. This is because laboratories developed values for the "normal range" by measuring hormone blood values of healthy women without knowledge of the women's sexual function. Thus the so-called "normal range" includes women who may not have been sexually healthy. Several studies have now examined the blood test values where women with sexual health concerns were excluded. These studies supported the consensus that if a hormone blood level falls in the lowest fourth or quartile of the current "normal range," it is considered suspicious. Another controversy is that blood test values may not represent what is actually happening inside the tissues.

When bothered by the clinical symptoms, and androgen blood test values are consistent with a hormonal problem, androgen treatment may be considered. The two most widely used androgens for treatment of sexual health problems are dehydroepiandrosterone and testosterone.

Dehydroepiandrosterone is not approved specifically for use in women with sexual health concerns, and therefore it is considered as "off-label" treatment. Your healthcare provider should inform you of this "off-label" use, and provide you with appropriate evidence-based information on risks and benefits. Each patient will then be better able to make an educated decision as to the potential use of this "off-label" medication.

The bioidentical (the same dehydroepiandrosterone molecule that your body synthesizes) form of dehydroepiandrosterone is available and recommended. It is usually obtained from a health food or vitamin store, however, it must be noted that the manufacturing standards for products from these stores are not consistent with those of FDA approved medications. It has been reported that many dehydroepiandrosterone products actually have limited amounts of active medication in the delivery system. The individual dose is best established by repeated follow-up blood tests of dehydroepiandrosterone-sulfate, usually at 6 week to 3-month intervals, until an appropriate blood level is stabilized.

In a small study, Arlt and co-investigators reported that use of dehydroepiandrosterone in women with sexual dysfunction and adrenal problems was associated with significant improvement in sexual function compared to those women who took placebo (sugar pills). Baulieu and colleagues found that dehydroepiandrosterone treatment approximately doubled serum total testosterone concentration, and also significantly increased skin hydration and bone density. Sexual interest was increased after 6 months of treatment, and sexual activity and sexual satisfaction were increased after 12 months. Recent publications by Davis and co-workers stressed that in pre-menopausal women, dehydroepiandrosterone-sulfate was the most representative androgen blood test value reflecting a problem with sexual health.

The most popular "off-label" androgen prescribed for treatment of sexual dysfunction in women is testosterone, used when bothersome clinical symptoms of androgen deficiency exist and "unbound" testosterone is low. There does not exist any FDA-approved pharmacologic treatment for women with sexual health problems in the United States. The testosterone patch has been approved in Europe by the EMEA for use in women with low desire following surgical menopause. From the perspective of androgen treatment, this means that the safety and/or efficacy data concerning use of androgens in a specific population of women with sexual health problems has been satisfactorily established at the time of publication of this book by the EMEA but not the FDA. There are FDA-approved versions of testosterone indicated for men for the treatment of hypogonadism. Use of these products in women with sexual health problems would be considered as an "off-label" treatment. As above, it is the responsibility of the healthcare clinician to provide you with appropriate evidence-based information on risks and benefits so an informed decision can be made. The individual dose for women with sexual health problems is usually 10% of a man's daily dose. It is important to repeat follow-up blood tests of "unbound" testosterone, usually at 3-month intervals, to establish the unique individual dose for each woman with sexual health concerns.

Although data supporting treatment of women with testosterone was limited until recently, reports documenting facilitation of the sexual response were published as early as 1938 by Shorr et al., in 1940 by Loeser, and in 1943 by Salmon and Geist. Even at that time it was appreciated by some that women's sexual function had a biological component, and that appropriate management involved attention to biological and psychological concerns.

There have been multiple double-blind, placebo-controlled studies of testosterone in women with sexual health concerns showing the benefits of testosterone use. The reader should be aware that of all the management strategies available to women for sexual dysfunction, including sex therapy, physical therapy, lifestyle modification, use of lubricants and devices, and change of medications, the evidence supporting these strategies is quite limited. Testosterone currently is the therapy most supported by evidence, although more research is needed.

In one study, post-menopausal women with sexual dysfunction randomized to testosterone treatment had significantly more satisfying sexual events, improved frequency of sexual activity, and improved sexual orgasm and pleasure compared to the placebo group. In another study of post-menopausal women, testosterone treatment was associated with significant improvement in a number of secondary sexual function outcome measures, including sexual arousal, orgasm, pleasure, and body image. Women assigned to testosterone also reported decreased concern or distress about sexual functioning. In a study of pre-menopausal women, those who received testosterone had significantly improved sexual motivation, fantasy, frequency of sexual activity, pleasure, orgasm, and satisfaction. Testosterone also significantly improved their scores on a validated wellbeing questionnaire.

According to the Princeton Consensus conference in 2001, it is recommended that women suspected of having androgen insufficiency be managed with systemic estrogen administration prior to starting androgen therapy with testosterone. Despite these recommendations, however, many women express reluctance to use exogenous estrogen due to fears and concerns of breast cancer, heart attack, and stroke, based on WHI data. Some women consider starting directly on androgen therapy to avoid the potential risks associated with exogenous estrogen use.

There is evidence that androgens are efficacious without concomitant estrogens in post-menopausal women with hypoactive sexual desire disorder. During a recent international sexual medicine meeting, 24 week data were presented concerning 771 post-menopausal women with hypoactive sexual desire disorder not receiving systemic estrogen therapy. The women were enrolled in a randomized, double-blind, multi-national study to evaluate the safety and efficacy of testosterone. Compared to placebo, testosterone (300 υg/day) significantly improved the 4-week frequency of multiple domains of the profile of female sexual function including satisfying sexual events and sexual desire, and significantly decreased distress. Mean testosterone levels and free testosterone levels at 6 months with the 300 υg/day testosterone were within the reference range for normal pre-menopausal women. There were no clinically significant changes in lab parameters measured over 24 weeks.

The long-term safety of testosterone use in women for sexual health concerns has not yet been established. Women considering treatment with testosterone for their sexual health concerns need to be aware of the following possible healthcare risks.

Concerning hirsutism (body hair growth) and acne, 3% to 8% of women users of testosterone for management of sexual health problems noted side effects. These side effects are usually mild and dependent upon dose and duration of testosterone treatment. Virilization (voice deepening, excessive growth of the clitoris, and scalp hair recession) is a targeted effect of the high testosterone doses used for management of female to male transsexuals (10 times the dose used for treatment of female sexual dysfunction).

Concerning breast cancer, the vast majority of reports show no increase in breast cancer risk among women using testosterone for management of sexual health problems. Of interest, there is no increased risk of breast cancer in women who have long-term elevated testosterone from polycystic ovary disease. Breast cancer potential was measured in monkeys using an index of breast tissue proliferation. In those treated with estradiol alone, the breast tissue proliferation was 4 times the control animals. In those animals co-treated with estradiol and testosterone, the risk was one half of the estradiol alone treated group. In a breast cancer comparison study, the cases of breast cancer per 100,000 women-years in women using estrogen and testosterone or estrogen, progesterone, and testosterone were lower than in women using estrogen and progesterone. Of note, whereas many studies show no increase in breast cancer in women using bioidentical testosterone, a recent study of nurses showed that those who used the non-bioidentical form of testosterone called methyl testosterone in conjunction with a fixed dose of estradiol did indeed have a higher risk of breast cancer compared to those who did not use the non-bioidentical form of testosterone.

Concerning the side effects of growth of the uterine lining, liver function changes, sleep apnea, and aggression, studies indicate these are not associated with use of the recommended doses of testosterone for women with sexual dysfunction.

What is the bottom line? Testosterone is a sex steroid critical for sexual function and structure in men and women. Safety and efficacy data with the judicious use of bioidentical testosterone are ongoing and available for all patients (and partners) and healthcare providers to analyze. Decisions based on risks and benefits for use of this sex steroid when androgen insufficiency exists will be individual. For those who decide the benefits outweigh the risks, the most prudent plan is to use bioidentical testosterone in doses that maintain hormone values in an appropriate physiologic range, have frequent and regular blood testing, and undergo annual breast exams, mammograms, and gynecologic exams. More research is needed.

References for Androgen Therapy:

Arlt W, Callies F, van Vlijmen JC, Koehler I, Reincke M, Bidlingmaier M, Huebler D, Oettel M, Ernst M, Schulte HM, Allolio B. Dehydroepiandrosterone replacement in women with adrenal insufficiency. N Engl J Med. 1999;341:1013–20. Annotation: Women with adrenal insufficiency received dehydroepiandrosterone orally each morning for 4 months and placebo daily for 4 months, with a 1-month washout period. Treatment with dehydroepiandrosterone raised the serum concentrations of dehydroepiandrosterone sulfate and testosterone into the normal range. serum concentrations of sex hormone binding globulin decreased significantly. Dehydroepiandrosterone significantly improved overall wellbeing as well as scores for depression and anxiety. As compared with placebo, dehydroepiandrosterone significantly increased the frequency of sexual thoughts, sexual interest, and satisfaction with both mental and physical aspects of sexuality.

Bachmann G, Bancroft J, Braunstein G, Burger H, Davis S, Dennerstein L, Goldstein I, Guay A, Leiblum S, Lobo R, Notelovitz M, Rosen R, Sarrel P, Sherwin B, Simon J, Simpson E, Shifren J, Spark R, Traish A; Princeton. Female androgen insufficiency: the Princeton consensus statement on definition, classification, and assessment. Fertil Steril. 2002;77:660–5. Annotation: This international consensus conference, known as the Princeton Conference, was assembled to evaluate androgen insufficiency as a cause of sexual problems in women. The result of the conference was a new term, "female androgen insufficiency," along with consensus-based guidelines for clinical assessment and diagnosis.

Baulieu EE, Thomas G, Legrain S, Lahlou N, Roger M, Debuire B, Faucounau V, Girard L, Hervy MP, Latour F, Leaud MC, Mokrane A, Pitti-Ferrandi H, Trivalle C, de Lacharriere O, Nouveau S, Rakoto-Arison B, Souberbielle JC, Raison J, Le Bouc Y, Raynaud A, Girerd X, Forette F. Dehydroepiandrosterone (DHEA), DHEA sulfate, and aging: contribution of the DHEAge Study to a sociobiomedical issue. Proc Natl Acad Sci USA. 2000;97:4279–84. Annotation: Women and men 60–79 years old were given dehydroepiandrosterone or placebo daily for a year in a double-blind, placebo-controlled study. No potentially harmful accumulation of dehydroepiandrosterone-sulfate and active steroids were recorded. Bone turnover improved selectively in women >70 years old. A significant increase in most sexual interest parameters was also found in these older women. Improvement of skin status was observed, particularly in terms of hydration, epidermal thickness, sebum production, and pigmentation.

Bell RJ, Donath S, Davison SL, Davis SR. Endogenous androgen levels and well-being: differences between premenopausal and postmenopausal women. Menopause. 2006;13:65–71. Annotation: A total of 621 pre-menopausal women from the community provided a morning blood sample and completed the Psychological General Well Being Index questionnaire on the same day. Dehydroepiandrosterone sulfate levels were independently and positively associated with the domain score for vitality.

Braunstein GD, Sundwall DA, Katz M, Shifren JL, Buster JE, Simon JA, Bachman G, Aguirre OA, Lucas JD, Rodenberg C, Buch A, Watts NB. Safety and efficacy of a testosterone patch for the treatment of hypoactive sexual desire disorder in surgically menopausal women: a randomized, placebo-controlled trial. Arch Intern Med. 2005;165:1582–9. Annotation: A 24-week, randomized, double-blind, placebo-controlled, parallel-group, multi-center trial was conducted in women aged 24–70 years who developed distressful low sexual desire after surgical removal of the ovaries and uterus, and who were receiving oral estrogen therapy. Compared with placebo, women receiving the 300 ʋg testosterone patch had significantly greater increases from baseline in sexual desire and in frequency of satisfying sexual activity. Adverse events occurred with similar frequency in both groups; no serious safety concerns were observed.

Burgess HE, Shousha S. An immunohistochemical study of the long-term effects of androgen administration on female-to-male transsexual breast: a comparison with normal female breast and male breast showing gynaecomastia. J Pathol. 1993;170:37–43. Annotations: The prevalence of normal acini and ducts, fibrosis, cysts, and apocrine metaplasia in transsexual specimens was not statistically different from that seen in normal controls. It is concluded that long-term androgen administration does not appear to have any significant lasting effect on the normal human female breast.

Davis SR, Davison SL, Donath S, Bell RJ. Circulating androgen levels and self-reported sexual function in women. JAMA. 2005;294:91–6. Annotation: Low sexual responsiveness for women aged 45 years or older was associated with higher odds of having a serum dehydroepiandrosterone-sulfate level below the 10th percentile for this age group. For women aged 18–44 years, having low sexual desire, low sexual arousal, and low sexual responsiveness was associated with having a dehydroepiandrosterone-sulfate level below the 10th percentile.

Davis SR, van der Mooren MJ, van Lunsen RH, Lopes P, Ribot J, Rees M, Moufarege A, Rodenberg C, Buch A, Purdie DW. Efficacy and safety of a testosterone patch for the treatment of hypoactive sexual desire disorder in surgically menopausal women: a randomized, placebo-controlled trial. Menopause. 2006;13:387–96. Annotation: The efficacy and safety of a testosterone patch was investigated in surgically menopausal women receiving concurrent transdermal estrogen. The testosterone-treated group experienced a significantly greater change from baseline in the domain sexual desire score compared with placebo. The domain scores for arousal, orgasm, decreased sexual concerns, responsiveness, and self-image, as well as decreased distress, were also significantly greater with testosterone therapy than placebo. Adverse events occurred with similar frequency in both groups, and no serious risks of therapy were observed.

Dimitrakakis C, Zhou J, Wang J, Belanger A, LaBrie F, Cheng C, Powell D, Bondy C. A physiologic role for testosterone in limiting estrogenic stimulation of the breast. Menopause. 2003;10:292–8. Annotation: Concomitant administration of a physiological dose of testosterone and standard estrogen therapy almost completely attenuates estrogen-induced increases in mammary epithelial proliferation in the ovariectomized monkey, suggesting that the increased breast cancer risk associated with estrogen treatment could be reduced by testosterone supplementation. These findings suggest that treatment with a balanced formulation including all ovarian hormones may prevent or reduce estrogenic cancer risk in the treatment of women with ovarian failure.

Dimitrakakis C, Jones RA, Liu A, Bondy CA. Breast cancer incidence in post-menopausal women using testosterone in addition to usual hormone therapy. Menopause. 2004;11:531–5. Annotation: This was a retrospective, observational study that followed 508 post-menopausal women receiving testosterone in addition to usual hormone therapy. Breast cancer status was ascertained by mammography at the initiation of testosterone treatment and biannually thereafter. There were seven cases of invasive breast cancer in this population of testosterone users, for an incidence of 238 per 100,000 woman-years. The rate for estrogen/progestin and testosterone users was 293 per 100,000 woman-years—substantially less than women receiving estrogen/progestin in the Women's Health Initiative study (380 per 100,000 woman-years) or in the "Million Women" Study (521 per 100,000 woman-years). The breast cancer rate in the testosterone users was closest to that reported for hormone therapy never-users in the latter study (283 per 100,000 woman-years), and their age-standardized rate was the same as for the general population. These observations suggest that the addition of testosterone to conventional hormone therapy for post-menopausal women does not increase and may indeed reduce the hormone therapy-associated breast cancer risk, thereby returning the incidence to the normal rates observed in the general, untreated population.

Giraldi A, Marson L, Nappi R, Pfaus J, Traish AM, Vardi Y, Goldstein I. Physiology of female sexual function: animal models. J Sex Med. 2004;1:237–53. Annotation: Sex steroid hormones, estrogens and androgens, are critical for structure and function of genital tissues including regulation of blood flow, lubrication, smooth muscle function, mucous production, and sex steroid receptor expression in genital tissues.

Graziottin A, Leiblum S. Biological and psychosocial etiology of female sexual dysfunction during the menopausal transition. J Sex Med. 2005;2:S133–45. Annotation: Menopause is associated with physiological and psychological changes that contribute to lower self-esteem, diminished sexual responsiveness, and sexual desire. The primary biological change is a decrease in circulating estrogen levels, initially accounting for diminished vaginal lubrication, while the age-dependent decline in testosterone and androgen function, starting in a woman's early 20's, may precipitate or exacerbate aspects of female sexual dysfunction.

Hatzichristou D, Rosen RC, Broderick G, Clayton A, Cuzin B, Derogatis L, Litwin M, Meuleman E, O'Leary M, Quirk F, Sadovsky R, Seftel A. Clinical evaluation and management strategy for sexual dysfunction in men and women. J Sex Med. 2004;1:49–57. Annotation: Three concepts underlie sexual medicine management: use of a patient-centered framework, use of evidence-based medicine, and use of a step-care management approach. When taken together, these three principles provide a balanced and integrated approach to sexual dysfunction management.

Loeser A. Subcutaneous implantation of female and male hormone in tablet form in women. BMJ. 1940;1:479–82. Annotation: Loeser reported that women treated with testosterone experienced increased sexual drive even among the older population. Enlargement of the clitoris was also noticed in some. Women treated with testosterone showed temporary occurrence of facial acne that disappeared after some time. Women on testosterone also acknowledged a feeling of wellbeing, more balanced moods, clear thinking, and some professed greater determination.

Nappi R, Salonia A, Traish AM, van Lunsen RHW, Vardi Y, Kodiglu A, Goldstein I. Clinical biologic pathophysiologies of women's sexual dysfunction. J Sex Med. 2005;2:4–25. Annotation: This manuscript summarizes the available evidence-based literature concerning hormonal, neurologic, and vascular organic pathophysiologies of women's sexual dysfunctions.

Pessina MA, Hoyt RF Jr, Goldstein I, Traish AM. Differential effects of estradiol, progesterone, and testosterone on vaginal structural integrity. Endocrinology. 2006;147:61–9. Annotation: This study demonstrates that estradiol and testosterone have differential effects on vaginal tissue, and that testosterone and estradiol hormones are critical for the maintenance of genital tissue structure.

Salmon U and Geist SH. Effects of androgens upon libido in women. J. Clin. Endo. 1943;3:235–38. Annotation: Androgens were postulated to have three actions in women: increase the susceptibility to psychosexual stimulation, increase the sensitivity of external genitalia, and increase the intensity of sexual gratification. Androgens in the normal mature woman may act as physiological sensitizers of both the psychic and somatic components of the sexual mechanism. It is imperative that the scientific and medical communities work together to develop better understanding of the physiology and pathophysiology of androgens in women's sexual function and dysfunction in order to better manage patients with complaints of sexual dysfunction.

Shilkaitis A, Green A, Punj V, Steele V, Lubet R, Christov K. Dehydroepiandrosterone inhibits the progression phase of mammary carcinogenesis by inducing cellular senescence via a p16-dependent but p53-independent mechanism. Breast Cancer Res. 2005;7:R1132–40. Annotation: Dehydroepiandrosterone induced a dose-dependent decrease in tumor burden. Dehydroepiandrosterone can suppress mammary carcinogenesis by altering various cellular functions.

Shorr E, Papanicolaou GN, Stimmel BF. Neutralization of ovarian follicular hormone in women by simultaneous administration of male sex hormone. Proc. Soc. Exptl. Bio. Med. 1938;38:759–62. Annotation: The action of androgens in women's sexual interest was first noted by Shorr in 1938 as an incidental finding in studies on the effects of androgens on menopause.

Somboonporn W, Davis SR. Testosterone effects on the breast: implications for testosterone therapy for women. Endocr Rev. 2004;25:374–88. Annotation: In experimental studies, androgens exhibit growth-inhibitory effects in some, but not all, breast cancer cell lines. In rodent breast cancer models, androgen action is anti-proliferative, despite the potential for testosterone and dehydroepiandrosterone to be aromatized to estrogen. The results from studies in rhesus monkeys suggest that testosterone may serve as a natural endogenous protector of the breast, and limit mitogenic and cancer-promoting effects of estrogen on mammary epithelium. The strongest data for exogenous testosterone therapy comes from primate studies. Based on such simulations, inclusion of testosterone in post-menopausal estrogen-progestin regimens has the potential to ameliorate the stimulating effects of combined estrogen-progestin on the breast.

Studd J, Bouchard C, Kroll R, Koch H, von Schoultz B, Davis S. The effect of a testosterone transdermal patch on hypoactive sexual desire disorder in postmenopausal women not receiving systemic estrogen therapy: The APHRODITE Study. J Sex Med. 2007;4:S112. Annotation: A recent randomized, double-blind, multinational study evaluated testosterone treatment in 771 menopausal women with hypoactive sexual desire disorder not receiving systemic estrogen and/or progesterone therapy. Testosterone significantly improved 4-week frequency of satisfying sexual activity, sexual desire, and multiple other domains of the profile of female sexual function, and decreased distress, versus placebo. Overall, adverse events and adverse event withdrawals were similar in the placebo and treated groups. There was no increase in the frequency of unwanted hair observed in the treated versus placebo group.

Tamimi RM, Hankinson SE, Chen WY, Rosner B, Colditz GA. Combined estrogen and testosterone use and risk of breast cancer in postmenopausal women. Arch Intern Med. 2006;166:1483–9. Annotation: The relation between the use of estrogen and testosterone therapies and breast cancer was evaluated. Among women with a natural menopause, the risk of breast cancer was nearly 2.5-fold greater among current users of estrogen plus methyltestosterone therapy than among never users.

Traish AM, Kim N, Min K, Munarriz R, Goldstein I. Role of androgens in female genital sexual arousal: receptor expression, structure, and function. Fertil Steril. 2002;77(Suppl 4):S11–8. Annotation: Observations are presented that androgens play an important role in modulating the physiology of vaginal tissue and contribute to peripheral genital sexual arousal.

Traish AM, Kim NN, Munarriz R, Moreland R, Goldstein I. Biochemical and physiological mechanisms of female genital sexual arousal. Arch Sex Behav.

2002;31:393–400. Annotation: This manuscript reviews research efforts from a number of laboratories in which several experimental models have been established, and concludes that understanding of the physiologic aspects of female sexual function is complex and requires investigation of vascular, neurological (central and peripheral), hormonal, and structural components.

Dopamine Agonist Therapy

Brain regulation of sexual behavior is complex and poorly understood, however it is evident that sexual behavior is modulated by a number of central nervous system neurotransmitters including dopamine. The activation of dopamine receptors may be a key intermediary, along with sex steroids, androgens, estrogens, and progestins, in the stimulation of central sexual arousal, desire, excitation, mood, and incentive-related sexual behavior. Clinical use of dopamine agonists has been reported to improve sexual function. The belief is that the increased brain levels of dopamine from dopamine agonists facilitate sexual functions, such as sexual interest and orgasm.

Bupropion is a widely used FDA-approved dopamine agonist for treatment of depression. It has fewer reported adverse sexual side effects than traditional selective serotonin reuptake inhibitor based anti-depressants. Bupropion appears to affect the uptake of two chemicals in the brain, dopamine and norepinephrine. In general, the "off-label" clinical use of buproprion in women with sexual dysfunction has been for low sexual desire and for anti-depressant-associated sexual dysfunction.

As it concerns women with hypoactive sexual desire disorder, the bupropion effect on the dopamine neurotransmitter system is considered prosexual. In one study of pre-menopausal women with low desire, compared to placebo, bupropion resulted in increased scores on a validated questionnaire for sexual pleasure, arousal, and orgasm. In a multi-site, single-blind study of pre-menopausal women with low desire, one-third of the women noted increased sexual interest. In another placebo-controlled trial, bupropion produced an increase in desire and frequency of sexual activity compared with placebo, however, frequency was correlated to total testosterone level at baseline and during treatment.

As it concerns women with sexual side effects from selective serotonin reuptake inhibitors, many antidotes have been proposed but few have been subjected to appropriate study. Some evidence has suggested that bupropion may be an effective antidote for selective serotonin reuptake inhibitor-induced sexual dysfunction. In a large study of patients with depression and normal sexual functioning, the incidence of orgasm problems and worsened sexual functioning was significantly lower with bupropion than with selective serotonin reuptake inhibitor. In another study of those with major depressive disorder receiving a selective serotonin reuptake inhibitor, sexual functioning improved after addition of bupropion. The improvement in sexual function continued with bupropion treatment alone after discontinuation of the selective serotonin reuptake inhibitor. In an additional study, bupropion improved sexual desire and frequency of sexual activity. Compared with selective serotonin reuptake inhibitors, bupropion revealed less desire dysfunction and less orgasm dysfunction and superior overall satisfaction with sexual functioning.

Another dopamine agonist is cabergoline, a drug that raises brain dopamine and lowers prolactin (an inhibitory central neurotransmitter) levels. Cabergoline can increase sexual interest and sexual orgasm, in part, by its dopamine agonist actions. Treatment with cabergoline, a potent and long-lasting dopamine agonist, is of particular benefit in the presence of high blood levels of prolactin. One study noted that cabergoline reversed sexual dysfunction in patients with high prolactin after 6 months of treatment. Cabergoline has also been used for sexual dysfunction not related to high prolactin. In patients with psychogenic sexual dysfunction, cabergoline treatment improved sexual desire, orgasmic function, and patient and partner sexual satisfaction.

In summary, dopamine agonist pharmacologic agents, such as bupropion and cabergoline, may be helpful in patients with sexual dysfunction. Currently, multiple dopamine agonist-like drugs are being studied in clinical investigations. It is likely that the future of pharmacologic management of sexual dysfunction in women will be in the development of central neurotransmitters including dopamine agonist-like agents.

References for Dopamine Agonist Therapy:

Beharry RK, Hale TM, Wilson EA, Heaton JP, Adams MA. Evidence for centrally initiated genital vasocongestive engorgement in the female rat: findings from a new model of female sexual arousal response. Int J Impot Res. 2003;15:122–8. Annotation: Dopamine receptor D_1/D_2 agonist apomorphine-induced behavioral and genital responses were characterized. Apomorphine stimulated a reproducible sexual arousal response in female rats involving obvious genital vasocongestive engorgement. Apomorphine-induced genital arousal responses are hormonally regulated and are markedly diminished by ovariectomy.

Clayton AH, McGarvey EL, Abouesh AI, Pinkerton RC. Substitution of an SSRI with bupropion sustained release following SSRI-induced sexual dysfunction. J Clin Psychiatry. 2001;62:185–90. Annotation: A total of 11 adults (8 women and 3 men) had major depressive disorder and were receiving a selective serotonin reuptake inhibitor. Depression and sexual dysfunction were assessed after bupropion SR was added to the current anti-depressant. Sexual functioning improved. Bupropion, as a therapy for depression, alleviates sexual dysfunction due to selective serotonin reuptake inhibitor treatment. Results show that sexual functioning improves after the addition of bupropion SR to selective serotonin reuptake inhibitor treatment and continues to improve, after discontinuation of the selective serotonin reuptake inhibitor, with bupropion SR treatment alone.

Clayton AH, Croft HA, Horrigan JP, Wightman DS, Krishen A, Richard NE, Modell JG. Bupropion extended release compared with escitalopram: effects on sexual functioning and antidepressant efficacy in 2 randomized, double-blind, placebo-controlled studies. J Clin Psychiatry. 2006;67:736–46. Annotation: A total of 830 adults with major depressive disorder participated. The incidence of orgasmic dysfunction and the incidence of worsened sexual functioning were statistically significantly lower with bupropion than with escitalopram, not statistically different between bupropion and placebo, and statistically significantly higher with escitalopram than with placebo. In one study, the percentage of patients with orgasmic dysfunction was 13% with bupropion, 32% with escitalopram, and 11% with placebo. In the other study, the respective percentages of patients with worsened sexual functioning at the end of the treatment period was 18% with bupropion, 37%, with escitalopram, and 14% with placebo. Bupropion had a sexual tolerability profile significantly better than that of escitalopram.

Dobkin RD, Menza M, Marin H, Allen LA, Rousso R, Leiblum SR. Bupropion improves sexual functioning in depressed minority women: an open-label switch study. J Clin Psychopharmacol. 2006;26:21–6. Annotation: This study of 18 depressed women was the first to examine a medication switch from a selective serotonin reuptake inhibitor to bupropion looking at sexual functioning. There were significant improvements in desire, arousal, and orgasm.

Fabre-Nys C, Chesneau D, de la Riva C, Hinton MR, Locatelli A, Ohkura S, Kendrick KM. Biphasic role of dopamine on female sexual behaviour via D2 receptors in the mediobasal hypothalamus. Neuropharmacology. 2003;44:354–66. Annotation: Dopamine has been implicated in the control of sexual behavior, but its role seems quite complex and controversial. Dopamine acts via D_2 receptors in the mediobasal hypothalamus of the brain to control female sexual behavior in a biphasic manner: the onset of sexual motivation and receptivity requiring an initial increase in activation followed by a decrease. This dual action could explain some of the controversies concerning dopamine action on sexual behavior.

Nickel M, Moleda D, Loew T, Rother W, Gil FP. Cabergoline treatment in men with psychogenic erectile dysfunction: a randomized, double-blind, placebo-controlled study. Int J Impot Res. 2006; doi:10.1038/sj.ijir.3901483. Annotation:

Cabergoline was studied in patients with psychogenic sexual dysfunction in a randomized, placebo-controlled, double-blind study. Cabergoline treatment resulted in improved sexual desire, orgasmic function, and the patient's and partner's sexual satisfaction.

Segraves RT, Clayton A, Croft H, Wolf A, Warnock J. Bupropion sustained release for the treatment of hypoactive sexual desire disorder in premenopausal women. J Clin Psychopharmacol. 2004;24:339–42. Annotation: Pre-menopausal women with hypoactive sexual desire disorder were studied in a randomized, double-blind, placebo-controlled trial of bupropion. All measures indicated greater sexual responsiveness in women receiving bupropion. There were significant increases in sexual arousal, orgasm, and sexual satisfaction.

Stafford SA, Coote JH. Activation of D2-like receptors induces sympathetic climactic-like responses in male and female anaesthetised rats. Br J Pharmacol. 2006;148:510–6. Annotation: Selective dopamine agonists and antagonists were used to investigate whether dopaminergic mechanisms influence the generation of ejaculatory-related responses. Administration of a mixed D_1 and D_2 receptor agonist, apomorphine, evoked the characteristic bursting pattern responses. Similar, but fewer, burst pattern responses could also be evoked by a selective D_2 and D_3 receptor agonist piribedil. In anesthetized female rats, a similar patterned bursting response occurred in response to apomorphine, suggesting a common neural mechanism may regulate sexual climactic reflexes in both sexes.

Estrogen Therapy

There are 3 different 18-carbon sex steroid estrogens, estrone (E_1), estradiol (E_2), and estriol (E_3). The most biologically relevant estrogen, as it concerns sexual health, is estradiol. Estrogen, similar to androgen, is required for normal structure and function of genital tissues. Estradiol in the blood passes into the genital cells (typically a smooth muscle cell for the genitals), acts on estrogen receptors in these genital cells, and induces the nucleus of these genital cells to synthesize proteins. The proteins direct messages to act on genital and other tissues to maintain structure and function. For example, an estrogenized vagina has a thick lining layer (epithelial layer) that is highly rugated or folded, a blood vessel-rich middle layer (lamina propria), and a substantial muscle layer (muscularis layer). During sexual arousal, an estrogenized vagina widens and lengthens, becomes lubricated, and has enhanced sensation. The vaginal pH is around 4 and, as such, provides great resistance to infections and discharge.

At menopause, the ovaries cease estradiol production. At some point after menopause, most women will have some degree of genital atrophy due to low estradiol values. Diminished estrogen production, consistent with menopause, is associated with thinning of all 3 layers of the vagina. There is diminished ability of the vagina to stretch during sexual arousal, and lubrication and sensitivity decrease. Vaginal dryness can lead to dyspareunia. Vaginal pH increases and inflammation, infections, and discharge are commonplace. The estrogen-deficient vagina is easily traumatized and can bleed during sexual activity or internal examination. Low estrogen also contributes to other genital changes, such as thinning of the hair of the mons and shrinkage of the labia minora. In addition, the labia majora flatten as the subcutaneous fat and elasticity of the structures diminish. Atrophic changes in many of the genital tissues can be detected within several months of an estrogen-reduced environment. Researchers found that vaginal dryness, burning, and dyspareunia were reported more often in women with levels of estradiol <50 pg/ml than in those with higher levels. Low estrogen values affect more than just sexual health: bone and skin health, sleep, mood, cognition, and many more metabolic and bodily functions.

There has been a great deal of controversy about the risks and benefits of estrogen therapy in peri-menopausal and post-menopausal women. Although your ovaries cease estradiol production at menopause, in some post-menopausal women, estrogen production continues in varying degrees through peripheral conversion of androgens to estrogen via the enzyme aromatase. Measuring blood level and assessing clinical history can determine if a post-menopausal woman still makes adequate estradiol for sexual health.

Estrogen therapy has been shown to lower vaginal pH, increase vaginal blood flow and lubrication, and restore clitoral and vaginal sensation. In an illustrative study, only 15% of women on systemic estrogen therapy reported vaginal dryness after a 5-year follow up, compared to 30% to 40% of those who did not use it. Dyspareunia, vaginal irritation, pain, dryness or burning were also observed less often among those who used systemic estrogen therapy, compared to those who did not. Relief from these vaginal atrophy symptoms can often lead to more sexual desire and sexual arousal.

Vaginal atrophy symptoms can be treated by local or systemic estrogen therapy. Local therapy can be delivered via vaginal estradiol creams, vaginal estradiol rings, and local vaginal estradiol tablets. While the vaginal lining is thin, which is typically during the first several weeks of application, a woman is particularly susceptible to systemic absorption of local estrogen, but this concern diminishes as the vaginal lining thickens. Local estradiol delivery systems are not designed to help systemic symptoms of menopause, such as hot flashes and night sweats.

Given the fact that there are different local estradiol delivery systems, each woman must determine which best suits her. Estradiol creams are considered by some women to be messy; intravaginal rings and tablets may be more convenient. The intravaginal ring is placed in the vagina every 3 months during which time it slowly releases estradiol into the local vaginal environment. One caveat of the intravaginal ring, however, is the need to fit in the individual's vagina and not be expelled if there is vaginal prolapse. A different option is the intravaginal estradiol tablet that is placed in the vagina several times per week with a special applicator. Another safe and effective local estrogen therapy is conjugated equine estrogen, however this non-bioidentical form of vaginal estradiol is unable to be measured in the blood. Many healthcare providers prefer bioidentical intravaginal estradiol, since blood levels of estradiol can be measured as a safety precaution. Estriol has also been used as a local estrogen therapy. This form of estrogen, associated with pregnancy, is not an FDA approved product and is only available through a compound pharmacy.

Local estrogen therapy with bioidentical estradiol can be as effective as systemic estrogen for treatment of specific vaginal atrophy symptoms. In fact, local estrogen therapy can restore the vaginal lining layer to its normal state within a short time period, usually within several weeks. Intravaginal estradiol can partly or completely restore vaginal health to that of pre-menopausal function, and improve or cure genital atrophy and dryness. Studies show estradiol released from a ring to have equivalent efficacy to estradiol in cream delivery form.

Concerning local vaginal estrogen therapy and its association with breast cancer, one study examined almost 1500 women with histologically confirmed breast cancer who used such treatments for bothersome vaginal symptoms. Local estrogen use did not result in an increased risk of recurrence of breast cancer.

Systemic estrogen therapy for treatment of vaginal atrophy symptoms can be oral or topical. Oral estrogens have been around for many years and have been the most common route of estrogen therapy. They are usually well tolerated and cost-effective. Systemic estrogen has been shown to significantly improve vasomotor symptoms, including hot flashes, night sweats, and sleep disturbance, all of which can impact a women's body image, mood, and sexual desire. Alleviation of such symptoms can often help increase both quality of life and satisfaction during sexual activity.

There are several drawbacks to the oral administration of estrogen, however. The drug must pass to the liver after being absorbed in the gastro-intestinal tract. This may increase the sex hormone binding globulin level and thus may act to reduce the amount of biologically active testosterone. The reduction in biologically active "unbound" testosterone in post-menopausal women on oral estrogen therapy is a common cause of decreased libido.

Transdermal topical estrogen therapy, in the form of a patch or gel, is an effective systemic treatment alternative to oral administration. It gets absorbed directly through the skin into the blood stream and thus may provide consistent blood estradiol levels. Transdermal estrogen therapy also avoids being absorbed in the gastro-intestinal tract and passing to the liver.

A new choice of systemic administration is through the vagina via a special vaginal ring administration designed for systemic absorption. The ring is placed intravaginally where it remains for 90 days. This ring has the added benefit of increasing both local and systemic estradiol levels.

All estrogens intended for systemic use can again be divided into bioidentical and non-bioidentical medications. Many healthcare providers prefer systemic bioidentical estradiol since blood levels can be measured as a safety precaution. One goal is to keep the values of estradiol in the post-menopausal woman at or around 50 pg/ml since researchers found less vaginal dryness, burning, and dyspareunia at this blood level compared to lower levels.

You have likely heard about the Women's Health Initiative (WHI) study. The use of systemic estrogen therapy in menopausal women declined abruptly as a result of that study. The Women's Health Initiative was designed to measure the rate of heart attacks in healthy post-menopausal women (on average 12 years post-menopause), with a mean of 64 years of age. Participants were divided into 2 groups, a non-bioidentical estrogen-progesterone arm for those with an intact uterus and a non-bioidentical estrogen only arm for women with prior hysterectomy. The non-bioidentical estrogen-progesterone arm studied the use of conjugated equine estrogen plus medroxyprogesterone acetate versus placebo, while the non-bioidentical estrogen only arm studied conjugated equine estrogen versus placebo. The Women's Health Initiative studies showed that the risks of non-bioidentical estrogen-progesterone therapy include breast cancer, heart attack, and stroke. Other risks of estrogen therapy include blood clots, deep vein thrombosis, and pulmonary embolus.

The data obtained from the Women's Health Initiative are based on the use of non-bioidentical estrogen therapy, conjugated equine estrogen with or without non-bioidentical progesterone, in an older population. The WHI data do not provide information for women considering bioidentical estradiol therapy in the peri-menopause or early post-menopause. The Women's Health Initiative trials tested only one drug regimen and did not provide information about the use of other estradiol doses, formulations, regimens, and routes of administration, or doses and duration of other estrogen therapies. In addition, because of non-bioidentical estradiol use, the WHI did not measure estradiol blood levels.

The North American Menopause Society's March 2007 position statement concerning hormone therapy for menopausal women states that for younger women who use estrogen and progestin to treat hot flashes, night sweats, and sexual dysfunctions, the benefits of short-term hormone treatment outweighed the risks. Younger women in the Women's Health Initiative study who were close to menopause when they used estrogen and progestin had an 11% lower risk of heart problems. On the other hand, older women, 20 years past menopause, had a 71% higher risk of heart attack. The WHI study also showed that the breast cancer risk for estrogen-only users was lower, with 8 fewer cancer cases per 10,000 women a year, and that the risk to an individual woman was low. Of note, women who used estrogen and progestin were 21% less likely to have diabetes mellitus.

However, the recent fear of estrogens has led many women to consider herbal therapies because they are advertised as "natural" and, by implication, "safer." Herbal therapies are not overseen by any government agency and the manufacturing is not regulated. What is on the label is not necessarily in the jar, and what is in the jar is not necessarily on the label. Numerous claims are made for these products, especially when it comes to sexual improvement effects. Women consumers should be wary about use of such products and of the claims of effect on sexual function. The basic principle is that the blood estradiol level is currently the most logical way of assessing the adequacy of estradiol therapy, herbal, prescription or otherwise.

In summary, estrogen use should be individualized to each woman's needs and expectations. There is no one formula for all women. What holds for women 10–20 years post-menopausal cannot be extrapolated to women recently post-menopausal. What holds for oral systemic estrogen therapy cannot be extrapolated to non-oral systemic estrogen therapy or to local vaginal estrogen therapy. As with all sexual healthcare concerns, consider seeking additional information from sexual healthcare professionals.

References for Estrogen Therapy:

Addis IB, Ireland CC, Vittinghoff E, Lin F, Stuenkel CA, Hulley S. Sexual activity and function in postmenopausal women with heart disease. Obstet Gynecol. 2005;106:121–7. Annotation: The Heart and Estrogen and Progestin Replacement Study (HERS) is a study of 2,763 post-menopausal women, average age 67 years, with coronary disease and intact uteri. Approximately 39% of the women in HERS were sexually active, and 65% of these reported at least 1 of 5 sexual problems (lack of interest, inability to relax, difficulty in arousal or in orgasm, and discomfort with sex). In multivariable analysis, factors independently associated with being sexually active included younger age, fewer years since menopause, being married, better self-reported health, higher parity, moderate alcohol use, not smoking, lack of chest discomfort, and not being depressed. Many women with heart disease continue to engage in sexual activity into their 70's; 2/3 of these report discomfort and other sexual function problems.

Anderson GL, Chlebowski RT, Rossouw JE, Rodabough RJ, McTiernan A, Margolis KL, Aggerwal A, David Curb J, Hendrix SL, Allan Hubbell F, Khandekar J, Lane DS, Lasser N, Lopez AM, Potter J, Ritenbaugh C. Prior hormone therapy and breast cancer risk in the Women's Health Initiative randomized trial of estrogen plus progestin. Maturitas. 2006;55:103–15. Annotation: A safe interval for combined hormone use could not be reliably defined. The increase in breast cancer risk in the overall trial, after only 5.6 years of follow-up, initially concentrated in women with prior hormone exposure, and then looked at increasing risk over time in women without prior exposure. Results suggest that durations only slightly longer than those in the Women's Health Initiative (WHI) trial are associated with increased risk of breast cancer.

Davey DA. Hormone replacement therapy: time to move on? Br Menopause Soc. 2006;12:75–80. Annotation: The risks and benefits of hormone replacement therapy need to be put in perspective. In the analyses of the Women's Health Initiative (WHI), the attributable risks were "appreciable" (i.e. more than 1/1000) only in women aged over 70 years, with the exception of the risks of venous thromboembolism and stroke. The women in the WHI trial do not represent the relatively younger, healthy, post-menopausal women most commonly prescribed hormone therapy, who are probably at much lower risk. Moreover, the WHI trial did not take into account the benefit of relief of menopausal symptoms that, for many women, outweigh the "rare" long-term risks.

Davis SR, Guay AT, Shifren JL, Mazer NA. Endocrine aspects of female sexual dysfunction. J Sex Med. 2004;1:82–6. Annotation: Various sex steroid hormones, including estrogen, progesterone, and testosterone, may influence female sexual function. Systemic estrogen or estrogen and progestin therapy may alleviate climacteric symptoms, but there is no evidence that this therapy specifically improves hypoactive sexual desire disorder in pre-menopausal or post-menopausal women. Exogenous testosterone has been shown in small, randomized, controlled trials to improve sexual desire, arousal, and sexual satisfaction in both pre-menopausal and post-menopausal women. Use of exogenous testosterone should be considered only after other causes of hypoactive sexual desire disorder have been excluded, such as depression, relationship problems, and poor health. Hormonal therapy should be individualized, risks and benefits fully discussed, and all treated women should be carefully monitored for therapeutic side effects.

Giraldi A, Marson L, Nappi R, Pfaus J, Traish AM, Vardi Y, Goldstein I. Physiology of female sexual function: animal models. J Sex Med. 2004;1:237–53. Annotation: Peripheral arousal states are dependent on regulation of genital smooth muscle tone. Sex steroid hormones, estrogens and androgens, are critical for structure and function of genital tissues, including modulation of genital blood flow, lubrication, neurotransmitter function, smooth muscle contractility, mucification, and sex steroid receptor expression in genital tissues.

Goldstein I, Alexander JL. Practical aspects in the management of vaginal atrophy and sexual dysfunction in perimenopausal and postmenopausal women. J Sex Med. 2005;2:S154–65. Annotation: Estrogen decline in peri- and post-menopause disrupts many physiological responses characteristic of sexual arousal, including smooth muscle relaxation, vasocongestion, and vaginal lubrication. Genital tissues depend on continued estrogen and androgen stimulation for normal function. An upward shift in vaginal pH, as the result of vaginal atrophy, alters the normal vaginal flora. Reduced lubrication capability and tissue elasticity, in addition to shortening and narrowing of the vaginal vault, can lead to painful and/or unpleasant intercourse. At the same time, diminished sensory response may reduce orgasmic intensity. Clinical management includes measures to enhance overall health, using topical or systemic hormone supplementation with estrogens and/or androgens. No single therapeutic approach is appropriate for every woman with peri- or post-menopausal sexual dysfunction; instead, treatment should be based on a comprehensive evaluation and consideration of medical and psychosocial contributors to the individual's dysfunction.

Graziottin A, Leiblum SR. Biological and psychosocial pathophysiology of female sexual dysfunction during the menopausal transition. J Sex Med. 2005;2: S133–45. Annotation: The primary biological change in menopause is a decrease in circulating estrogen levels. Estrogen deficiency initially accounts for irregular menstruation and diminished vaginal lubrication. Continual estrogen loss is associated with changes in the vascular, muscular, and urogenital systems, and also alterations in mood, sleep, and cognitive functioning, influencing sexual function both directly and indirectly. The age-dependent decline in testosterone and androgen function, starting in a woman's early 20's, may precipitate or exacerbate aspects of sexual dysfunction; these effects are most pronounced following bilateral ovariectomy and consequent loss of 50% or more of total testosterone. Non-hormonal factors that affect sexuality are health status and current medication use, changes in or dissatisfaction with partner, partner's health and/or sexual problems, and socioeconomic status.

Kovalevsky G. Female sexual dysfunction and use of hormone therapy in post-menopausal women. Semin Reprod Med. 2005;23:180–7. Annotation: Sexual dysfunction is a common problem for women of all ages and remains an important aspect of women's health following menopause. It appears that lack of estrogen may lead to sexual dysfunction, primarily by causing vaginal atrophy and dyspareunia. These symptoms may be treated by systemic or local estrogen therapy. Conversely, androgen insufficiency appears to be most strongly linked to diminished sexual desire. Growing evidence indicates that administration of androgens may be beneficial in such situations.

Nappi RE, Wawra K, Schmitt S. Hypoactive sexual desire disorder in postmenopausal women. Gynecol Endocrinol. 2006;22:318–23. Annotation: Decreases in sex hormone levels with menopause may result in consequences to women's general health and sexual wellbeing. In addition to the role of estrogens in preserving the biological basis of sexual response, there is emerging evidence that androgens are significant independent determinants affecting sexual desire, activity, and satisfaction, as well as mood and energy. While conventional hormone therapy with estrogens or estrogens and progestogens may be effective for vaginal atrophy, increasing vaginal lubrication, and reducing dyspareunia, many women with sexual dysfunction, especially low interest, remain unresponsive. In women on estrogen therapy, addition of testosterone resulted in significantly greater increases in satisfying sexual activity and sexual desire, and greater decreases in distress, than placebo-treated women.

North American Menopause Society. Estrogen and progestogen use in peri- and postmenopausal women: March 2007 position statement of The North American Menopause Society, Menopause. 2007;14:1–17. Annotation: The goal was to update the evidence-based position statement of the North American Menopause Society regarding recommendations for estrogen and progestogen use in peri- and post-menopausal women. The panel concluded that current evidence supports the use of estrogen therapy or estrogen and progestin therapy for menopause-related symptoms and disease prevention in appropriate populations of peri- and post-menopausal women.

Sarrel PM. Sexuality and menopause. Obstet Gynecol. 1990;75(Suppl 4):26S–30S. Annotation: Common sexual complaints include loss of desire, decreased frequency of sexual activity, painful intercourse, diminished sexual responsiveness, and dysfunctions of the male partner. Sexual function is influenced by biological and non-biological factors. Ovarian hormone levels can influence sexual arousal, including sensory perception, central and peripheral nerve discharge, peripheral blood flow, and the capacity to develop muscle tension, as well as sexual desire and frequency of sexual activity.

Sarrel PM. Effects of hormone replacement therapy on sexual psychophysiology and behavior in postmenopause. J Womens Health Gend Based Med. 2000;9: S25–32. Annotation: Dyspareunia due to vaginal dryness appears to be most responsive to estrogen therapy via restoration of vaginal cells, pH, and blood flow. Estrogen therapy has also been reported to enhance sexual desire in a significant percentage of women. Although treatment with estrogen therapy has been shown to be efficacious for many women, there are others whose sexual difficulties remain unresponsive. For some of these women, the addition of androgen has proved helpful.

Sarrel PM. Androgen deficiency: menopause and estrogen-related factors. Fertil Steril. 2002;77(Suppl 4):S63–7. Annotation: Estrogen depletion and replacement therapy at menopause can have clinically significant effects on bioavailability of endogenous androgens. Androgens complement the actions of estrogens in symptom control and disease prevention in post-menopausal women.

Stefanick ML, Anderson GL, Margolis KL, Hendrix SL, Rodabough RJ, Paskett ED, Lane DS, Hubbell FA, Assaf AR, Sarto GE, Schenken RS, Yasmeen S, Lessin L, Chlebowski RT. Effects of conjugated equine estrogens on breast cancer and mammography screening in postmenopausal women with hysterectomy. JAMA. 2006;295:1647–57. Annotation: Treatment with conjugated equine estrogens alone does not increase breast cancer incidence in post-menopausal women with prior hysterectomy. Initiation of conjugated equine estrogens should be based on consideration of the individual woman's potential risks and benefits.

Lubricants and Moisturizers

Vaginal lubricants and moisturizers are widely used by women of all ages with sexual health concerns. Vaginal lubricants are not exclusively for women in menopause. Vaginal dryness may occur during various parts of the menstrual cycle, during pregnancy, after childbirth, during nursing, at times of emotional stress and when the partner uses a condom. Various medications such as birth control pills, patches or rings, sleeping pills, anti-anxiety agents, anti-depressant agents, anti-hypertensive agents, and even cold and allergy medications can interfere with vaginal lubrication. Vaginal dryness may occur during intercourse if the woman is not sufficiently aroused and there is inadequate foreplay. Communication with the partner about what feels good is important. In addition, having intercourse more regularly may help promote enhanced vaginal lubrication. Pain disorders commonly reduce sexual arousal, thus reducing natural lubrication.

Physiologic treatments for vaginal dryness primarily involve use of local or systemic estrogen to the vagina, vestibule, and vulva to maximize genital structure and function. For women who cannot use estrogen therapy, non-estrogen vaginal lubricants and moisturizers used on a regular basis are an alternative. While these products do not treat the source of the problem, lubricants and moisturizers can be used successfully to manage vaginal itching, irritation, and dyspareunia. Furthermore, local use of vaginal lubricants can ease penetration and facilitate intercourse, and may help increase vaginal blood flow.

There are many different types of vaginal lubricants available over the counter that can lubricate the vagina for several hours. The product that works best for an individual is based on personal and partner preference. Vaginal lubricant delivery systems include vaginal suppositories, gels, creams, sprays, and edible forms. Lubricants should be pH neutral so the vaginal environment and flora are not altered. Water-based lubricants are easily absorbed; silicone-based lubricants leave the skin with an oily texture. It is critical to note, when that contraception is important, petroleum-based lubricants and oils decrease condom integrity. Vaginal lubricants are applied to the vaginal opening and to the partner's penis prior to penetration. Vaginal moisturizers can provide long-term relief of vaginal dryness, producing a longer duration of lubrication and a significantly lower vaginal pH than lubricants.

Vaginal lubricants and moisturizers are widely used by women without sexual health concerns to improve sexual satisfaction. Vaginal lubricants can also be used to enhance other sexual activities including masturbation with or without a vibrator, mutual masturbation, oral sex, and anal sex.

References for Lubricants and Moisturizers:

Amsterdam A, Carter J, Krychman M. Prevalence of psychiatric illness in women in an oncology sexual health population: a retrospective pilot study. J Sex Med. 2006;3:292–5. Annotation: A retrospective review was performed using 204 sequential charts of patients who attended the Sexual Health Program at Memorial Sloan-Kettering Cancer Center from March 2003 through August 2004. Among the most frequently encountered sexual complaints were dyspareunia (65%) and vaginal dryness (63%). Among the various treatment recommendations for sexual dysfunction, vaginal moisturizers and lubricants were widely used.

Johnston SL, Farrell SA, Bouchard C, Farrell SA, Beckerson LA, Comeau M, Johnston SL, Lefebvre G, Papaioannou A. The detection and management of vaginal atrophy. J Obstet Gynaecol Can. 2004;26:503–15. Annotation: A comprehensive approach to the discussion of available therapeutic and non-therapeutic options for vaginal atrophy was performed. Recommendations included: healthcare providers should routinely assess post-menopausal women for the symptoms and signs of vaginal atrophy, a common condition that exerts significant negative effects on quality of life; regular sexual activity should be encouraged to maintain vaginal health; vaginal moisturizers applied on a regular basis have an efficacy equivalent to local hormone replacement for the treatment of local urogenital symptoms such as vaginal itching, irritation, and dyspareunia, and should be offered to women wishing to avoid use of hormone therapy.

Leiblum SR. Arousal disorders in women: complaints and complexities. Med J Aust. 2003;178:638–40. Annotation: Female sexual arousal disorders constitute a varied spectrum of difficulties, ranging from the total absence of genital or subjective pleasurable arousal to feelings of persistent genital arousal in the absence of sexual desire. Arousal disorders can be associated with physical factors (e.g., vaginal dryness) or psychological factors (e.g., anxiety, distraction), or a combination of both. The most common complaint is the absence of subjective sexual excitement or pleasure despite adequate physical arousal (e.g., lubrication). Treatments include the use of lubricants.

Morali G, Polatti F, Metelitsa EN, Mascarucci P, Magnani P, Marre GB. Open, non-controlled clinical studies to assess the efficacy and safety of a medical device in form of gel topically and intravaginally used in postmenopausal women with genital atrophy. Arzneimittelforschung. 2006;56:230–8. Annotation: Menopause is often associated with vaginal atrophy and related symptoms, such as vaginal dryness, burning, itching, and sexual pain, and in general, a decrease in the quality of life. As an alternative to hormonal therapy, studies were performed to investigate the effects of a vaginal gel, with the aim of testing its safety and efficacy in post-menopausal women with urogenital atrophy. One study was carried out according to a multi-center, open, non-controlled design. A total of 100 post-menopausal women were assigned to the vaginal application of 2.5 g of gel/day for 1 week followed by 2 applications/week for 11 weeks. Results showed a marked effect of the gel on the vaginal dryness and on symptoms and signs with statistically significant reductions since the first week of treatment. No subjects complained of treatment-related adverse events, and the treatment course showed a high level of acceptability by the subjects.

Nieman LK. Management of surgically hypogonadal patients unable to take sex hormone replacement therapy. Endocrinol Metab Clin North Am. 2003;32:325–36. Annotation: In women, continued sexual intercourse and use of vaginal lubricants and moisturizers help to minimize symptoms of vaginal atrophy but do not ameliorate urinary symptoms.

Mediterranean Diet

There are peer-reviewed, evidence-based published data that metabolic syndrome affects sexual health, and therefore a change in eating habits, in particular to the Mediterranean diet that improves endothelial health, can positively influence the sexual health of women.

Contemporary women, in general, have decreased their physical activity and increased digestion of processed foods. The result has been an increase in metabolic syndrome, obesity, hypertension, high cholesterol, high blood levels of glucose, and diabetes. Man evolved from the hunter-gatherer caveman who ate fruit, nuts, berries, fish, and little meat, consistent with the current Mediterranean diet. The genetic material that existed in the caveman is the same genetic material that exists in contemporary times. The real life and health match, especially for vascular health, is the match of our genetic information with our ancestral diet, that is, the Mediterranean diet.

The Mediterranean diet reflects the eating habits traditionally followed by the people of the countries that border the Mediterranean Sea, and varies according to culture, ethnic background, and religion of the region. The hunter/gatherer diet must be supported by its active lifestyle; translated to modern times, at least 20 minutes per day of physical activity is critical. The diet consists of a high consumption of fruits, vegetables, potatoes, beans, nuts, seeds, breads, and other cereals relying on local, seasonal fresh produce. The contemporary Mediterranean diet utilizes olive oil widely for cooking and dressings, with a low to moderate amount of full fat cheese and yogurt. There is a modest consumption of wine, usually with meals, as well as a moderate amount of fish but little meat. An adequate intake of water must be maintained.

The key scientific finding is that the Mediterranean diet has been shown in placebo-controlled studies to lower endothelial inflammation, potentially contributing to the prevention of vascular diseases such as coronary heart disease. The reason for the Mediterranean diet lowering endothelial inflammation is not fully understood. Antioxidants and inducers of detoxification enzymes exist in abundance in vegetables, fruit, and virgin olive oil.

There are data that the Mediterranean diet lowers endothelial inflammation and reduces the prevalence of metabolic syndrome. A three-year study was conducted among men and women with metabolic syndrome. Men and women assigned to the Mediterranean diet were instructed to follow a Mediterranean-style diet and received detailed advice about how to increase daily consumption of whole grains, fruits, vegetables, nuts, and olive oil. Men and women consuming the Mediterranean diet had significantly reduced serum concentrations of multiple markers of endothelial cell inflammation, including C-reactive protein. In those individuals on the Mediterranean diet, the score of Endothelial Function improved. In those on the control diet, Endothelial Function scores remained elevated. At 2 years of follow-up, a significant number of men and women with metabolic syndrome on the Mediterranean diet and no other treatment were successfully managed and no longer met criteria for metabolic syndrome compared with subjects eating the control diet.

Are there data to support that the Mediterranean diet might be effective in reducing the prevalence of sexual dysfunction in men and women with metabolic syndrome? A 2-year study of men with metabolic syndrome and erectile dysfunction showed an improvement in the sexual function for the Mediterranean diet group. Another study compared pre-menopausal women with metabolic syndrome and sexual health problems with a control general population of women. Compared with the control group, women with metabolic syndrome and sexual dysfunction had lower total sexual function scores, lower sexual satisfaction scores, and higher markers of endothelial inflammation such as C-reactive protein. Thus, in women with metabolic syndrome, there is the same inverse relation of sexual function to markers of endothelial inflammation. Research is ongoing to see if women with metabolic syndrome and sexual health concerns who follow the Mediterranean diet will improve sexual function. Given the results in men, it appears that returning to the caveman days, eating and exercising more appropriately, makes good sense for sexual health as well as overall health.

References for Mediterranean Diet:

Davey DA. Hormone replacement therapy: time to move on? Br Menopause Soc. 2006;12:75–80. Annotation: The risks and benefits of hormone replacement therapy need to be put in perspective. In the analyses of the Women's Health Initiative (WHI), the attributable risks were "appreciable" (i.e. more than 1/1000) only in women aged over 70 years, with the exception of the risks of venous thromboembolism and stroke. The women in the WHI trial do not represent the relatively younger, healthy, post-menopausal women most commonly prescribed hormone therapy who are probably at much lower risk. Moreover, the WHI trial did not take into account the benefit of relief of menopausal symptoms that, for many women, outweigh the "rare" long-term risks.

Esposito K, Pontillo A, Di Palo C, Giugliano G, Masella M, Marfella R, Giugliano D. Effect of weight loss and lifestyle changes on vascular inflammatory markers in obese women: a randomized trial. JAMA. 2003;289:1799–804. Annotation: A total of 120 pre-menopausal obese women aged 20–46 years, without diabetes, hypertension or hyperlipidemia, participated in a randomized, single-blind trial using a low-energy Mediterranean-style diet. After 2 years, body mass index decreased more in the intervention group than in controls, as did serum concentrations of interleuken-6, interleuken-18, and C-reactive protein. A multidisciplinary program aimed to reduce body weight in obese women through lifestyle changes was associated with a reduction in markers of vascular inflammation.

Esposito K, Marfella R, Ciotola M, Di Palo C, Giugliano F, Giugliano G, D'Armiento M, D'Andrea F, Giugliano D. Effect of a mediterranean-style diet on endothelial dysfunction and markers of vascular inflammation in the metabolic syndrome: a randomized trial. JAMA. 2004;292:1440–6. Annotation: A total of 180 patients (81 women) with the metabolic syndrome participated in a randomized, single-blind trial. Those assigned to the intervention group were instructed to follow a Mediterranean-style diet of daily consumption of whole grains, fruits, vegetables, nuts, and olive oil. After 2 years, patients following the Mediterranean-style diet were observed to have significantly reduced serum concentrations of C-reactive protein, interleuken-6, interleuken-7, and interleuken-18, as well as decreased insulin resistance, compared to the control group. At 2 years, 40 patients in the intervention group still had features of the metabolic syndrome, compared with 78 patients in the control group.

Esposito K, Ciotola, M, Marfella, R, Di Tommaso, D, Cobellis, L, Giugliano, D. Sexual Dysfunction in Women With the Metabolic Syndrome. Diabetes Care. 2005;28:756. Annotation: The prevalence of sexual dysfunction in pre-menopausal women with the metabolic syndrome was compared with the general female population. Women with the metabolic syndrome were matched with women of the control group for age, height, and weight, as well as pre-menopausal state. Compared with the control group, women with the metabolic syndrome had a reduced mean total Female Sexual Function Index score and an increased prevalence of sexual dysfunctions.

Esposito K, Ciotola M, Marfella R, Di Tommaso D, Cobellis L, Giugliano D. The metabolic syndrome: a cause of sexual dysfunction in women. Int J Impot Res. 2005;17:224–6. Annotation: A total of 200 pre-menopausal women with the metabolic syndrome participated. Compared with the control group of 80 women, 120 women with the metabolic syndrome had significantly reduced mean Female Sexual Function Index scores, reduced satisfaction rate, and higher circulating levels of C-reactive protein.

Esposito K, Ciotola M, Giugliano F, De Sio M, Giugliano G, D'armiento M, Giugliano D. Mediterranean diet improves erectile function in subjects with the metabolic syndrome. Int J Impot Res. 2006;18:405–10. Annotation: Sixty-five men with the metabolic syndrome and erectile dysfunction met the inclusion/exclusion criteria; 35 were assigned to the Mediterranean-style diet, rich in whole grain, fruits, vegetables, legumes, walnuts, and olive oil, and 30 to the control diet. After 2 years, endothelial function score and inflammatory markers improved in the intervention group, but remained stable in the control group. A total of 13 men in the intervention group reported an International Index of Erectile Function score of 22 or higher.

Giugliano F, Esposito K, Di Palo C, Ciotola M, Giugliano G, Marfella R, D'Armiento M, Giugliano D. Erectile dysfunction associates with endothelial dysfunction and raised proinflammatory cytokine levels in obese men. J Endocrinol Invest. 2004;27:665–9. Annotation: A total of 80 obese men were divided into two groups according to the presence or absence of erectile dysfunction. Compared with non-obese age-matched men, obese men had higher circulating concentrations of the proinflammatory cytokines interleuken-6, interleuken-8, and interleuken-18, as well as C-reactive protein. C-reactive protein levels were significantly higher in obese men with erectile dysfunction, as compared with obese men without erectile dysfunction.

Miller EL, Mitchell A. Metabolic syndrome: screening, diagnosis, and management. J Midwifery Womens Health. 2006;51:141–51. Annotation: Metabolic syndrome is a cluster of health findings that increase the risk of cardiovascular events. The prevalence of metabolic syndrome is high in women and is linked to several conditions unique to women's health, including female sexual dysfunction.

Progesterone Therapy

Progesterone is a 21-carbon sex steroid. Like estrogen and testosterone, progesterone acts by entering the cell and binding to its own receptor in the cell. The combination of progesterone and receptor enters the nucleus to activate the synthesis of important proteins. It is thought that when progesterone acts in the brain, one of its roles is to regulate nerves that control sexual behavior. In a woman with an intact uterus, the addition of progesterone to estrogen therapy is needed to prevent thickening of the lining and possible cancer of the uterus. Progesterone appears to work by lowering the estrogen receptors in the lining of the uterus.

Progesterone or progestogens can be administered in daily doses. They can also be administered using several different cyclical regimens in which progesterone is taken during only a portion of the cycle, for example, the last 10–14 days of the hormone therapy cycle. Concerning the relative risk of endometrial cancer with hormone therapy, there was no difference found between continuous and intermittent progesterone regimens.

Bioidentical oral progesterone is absorbed from the gastrointestinal system and delivered via a micronization process in which the progesterone is broken down into small particles to help with its absorption. By using bioidentical progesterone, the healthcare professional is able to record progesterone blood levels. In contrast, there are numerous synthetic, non-bioidentical progestogens, some related to progesterone and some related to testosterone, but these cannot be measured in the blood.

In animal studies, use of bioidentical progesterone and bioidentical estradiol was associated with improved sexual mood and interest. This was in sharp contrast to the use of estradiol in combination with a synthetic non-bioidentical progestogen, where sexual mood and sexual interest were significantly reduced. More research is needed in this area.

References for Progesterone Therapy:

Brandling-Bennett EM, Blasberg ME, Clark AS. Paced mating behavior in female rats in response to different hormone priming regimens. Horm Behav. 1999;35:144–54. Annotation: A female rat will display a repertoire of behaviors during a sexual encounter with a male rat, including sexually receptive (the lordosis response) and proceptive (hopping, darting) behaviors. In addition, when given the opportunity, a sexually receptive female rat will approach and withdraw from the male rat, controlling the timing of the receipt of mounts, intromissions, and ejaculations, a behavior known as paced mating behavior. The present experiments tested the hypotheses that progesterone regulates paced mating behavior, and that multiple hormone regimens used previously to induce sexual receptivity have the same effect on paced mating behavior. The number of hops and darts per minute increased with the dose of progesterone administered.

Davis SR, Guay AT, Shifren JL, Mazer NA. Endocrine aspects of female sexual dysfunction. J Sex Med. 2004;1:82–6. Annotation: Various endogenous hormones, including progesterone, may influence female sexual function. Progestins appear to have little impact in either direction on the urogenital effects of estrogen, and have no proven benefit on other aspects of sexuality when given alone. Hormonal therapy should be individualized, with risks/benefits fully discussed, and all treated women should be carefully monitored for therapeutic side effects.

Giraldi A, Marson L, Nappi R, Pfaus J, Traish AM, Vardi Y, Goldstein I. Physiology of female sexual function: animal models. J Sex Med. 2004;1:237–53. Annotation: Proceptive behaviors are dependent, in part, on progesterone.

Molenda-Figueira HA, Williams CA, Griffin AL, Rutledge EM, Blaustein JD, Tetel MJ. Nuclear receptor coactivators function in estrogen receptor- and progestin receptor-dependent aspects of sexual behavior in female rats. Horm Behav. 2006;50:383-92. Annotation: The ovarian hormones, estradiol and progesterone, facilitate the expression of sexual behavior in female rats. While female sexual behaviors can be activated by high doses of estradiol alone in ovariectomized rats, the full repertoire of female sexual behavior, in particular hopping, darting, and ear wiggling, is considered to be progesterone dependent.

Pazol K, Wilson ME, Wallen K. Medroxyprogesterone acetate antagonizes the effects of estrogen treatment on social and sexual behavior in female macaques. J Clin Endocrinol Metab. 2004;89:2998–3006. Annotation: Medroxyprogesterone acetate is used commonly in contraception and hormone replacement therapy, however, little is known about its effects within the central nervous system. Treatment with estradiol alone induced a substantial rise in female sexual initiation rates. Natural progesterone treatment did not significantly inhibit sexual behavior. Medroxyprogesterone acetate treatment markedly antagonized estradiol's effects. These findings suggest that medroxyprogesterone acetate antagonizes certain behavioral effects of estradiol that may be beneficial to women, and that it does so more profoundly or in ways that endogenous progesterone does not.

Pazol K, Northcutt KV, Wilson ME, Wallen K. Medroxyprogesterone acetate acutely facilitates and sequentially inhibits sexual behavior in female rats. Horm Behav. 2006;49:105–13. Annotation: Medroxyprogesterone acetate, a synthetic progestin commonly used in contraception and hormone replacement therapy, appears to inhibit libido in women. The actions of medroxyprogesterone acetate and natural progesterone on sexual behavior in female rats were compared. Medroxyprogesterone acetate attenuated the expression of proceptive and receptive behavior at both the mid and high doses, whereas natural progesterone only attenuated the expression of lordosis and only did so at the highest dose.

Vasodilator Therapy

Basic science studies investigating the physiology of sexual function utilizing female animal models reveal that the same chemicals that are involved in the physiology of male erection are found in women's genital tissues, such as clitoral, vaginal, and labial tissues. Phosphodiesterase type 5 inhibitors, such as sildenafil (Viagra™), act on these chemicals and facilitate the erectile response in men. Can sildenafil-like drugs facilitate vasodilation and peripheral arousal physiology in women?

There have been several clinical studies on phosphodiesterase type 5 inhibitors over the last few years, conducted in either pre-menopausal or post-menopausal women with sexual health concerns, as well as in healthy women without sexual dysfunction. An important point in treating women with sexual health concerns is that a normal milieu of androgens and estrogens is needed to achieve benefits from sildenafil-like drugs. Many past studies of these drugs did not take into account the androgen and estrogen blood test values; the focus was on women with sexual health concerns without regard to their hormonal biochemistry. The reader is reminded that sex steroid hormones are required for structure and function of women's genital tissues. What was not appreciated at the time of the early studies was that phosphodiesterase type 5 inhibitor drugs require functional genital tissues to work. It is now well understood that these drugs do not work in men without normal testosterone values.

The following studies assessed safety and efficacy of phosphodiesterase type 5 inhibitor drugs in women with normal androgens and estrogens. A double-blind, crossover, placebo-controlled safety and efficacy study of sildenafil was performed in pre-menopausal women affected by female sexual arousal disorder who did not have problems with sexual interest and had normal levels of steroid hormones. Subjects were observed to benefit from treatment with the sildenafil showing improvement in sexual arousal, orgasm, frequency, and enjoyment of sexual intercourse versus placebo.

A double-blind, placebo-controlled safety and efficacy study with sildenafil was performed in post-menopausal women with female sexual arousal disorder who had adequate serum estradiol and testosterone values. Women with female sexual arousal disorder and no problems with sexual interest, who were assigned the active drug sildenafil, had a significantly greater improvement in sexual arousal, orgasm, intercourse, and overall satisfaction with sexual life, compared with placebo.

A randomized, double-blind, crossover, placebo-controlled safety and efficacy study with sildenafil was performed in pre-menopausal women asymptomatic for sexual disorders, with normal ovulatory cycles, and with normal levels of steroid hormones. Sildenafil improved general sexual behavior including sexual arousal, orgasm, and enjoyment versus placebo. The study suggested that phosphodiesterase type 5 inhibitors improve women's sexual experience.

Sildenafil has been studied as an antidote to psychotropic-induced sexual dysfunction in women. In one study, women reported significant improvements in all domains of sexual function, with improvement in overall sexual satisfaction after sildenafil treatment. Significant improvements were reported regardless of psychotropic medication type. Patients taking selective serotonin re-uptake inhibitors reported less improvement in arousal, libido, and overall sexual satisfaction than did other patients, whereas patients taking benzodiazepines (such as Valium) reported significantly more improvement in libido and overall sexual satisfaction.

Selective phosphodiesterase type 5 inhibitors seem to be effective in selected populations of pre-menopausal and post-menopausal women with sexual arousal disorder. Selection criteria best associated with success included having normal sex steroid hormonal milieu and no hypoactive sexual desire disorder. Selective phosphodiesterase type 5 inhibitors may have a role as an antidote to psychotropic-induced sexual dysfunction.

There are also topical vasodilators, such as prostaglandin E_1, to increase genital arousal. These products are currently under development, with studies ongoing. In a very small study of 10 woman, a non-prescription botanical feminine massage oil called Zestra for Women™ has shown promise in improving sexual pleasure and arousal when applied to the vulva.

References for Vasodilator Therapy:

Basson R, McInnes R, Smith MD, Hodgson G, Koppiker N. Efficacy and safety of sildenafil citrate in women with sexual dysfunction associated with female sexual arousal disorder. J Womens Health Gend Based Med. 2002;11:367–77. Annotation: A total of 577 estrogenized and 204 estrogen-deficient women with sexual dysfunction that included female sexual arousal disorder were randomized to treatment. Differences in efficacy between sildenafil and placebo were not significant for any patient or partner end points.

Bechara A, Bertolino MV, Casabe A, Fredotovich N. A double-blind randomized placebo control study comparing the objective and subjective changes in female sexual response using sublingual apomorphine. J Sex Med. 2004;1:209–14. Annotation: A total of 24 patients with orgasmic sexual dysfunction were included in a prospective, randomized, crossover protocol using 3 mg SL apomorphine. Compared to placebo, 3 mg SL apomorphine resulted in significantly higher clitoral blood flow and significantly increased sexual arousal and lubrication.

Caruso S, Intelisano G, Farina M, Di Mari L, Agnello C. The function of sildenafil on female sexual pathways: a double-blind, cross-over, placebo-controlled study. Eur J Obstet Gynecol Reprod Biol. 2003;110:201–6. Annotation: A total of 38 healthy women, asymptomatic for sexual disorders, participated. Sildenafil improved arousal, orgasm, and enjoyment with respect to placebo. Significant differences were noted during sildenafil usage with respect to the baseline for arousal, orgasm, and sexual enjoyment.

Caruso S, Agnello C, Intelisano G, Farina M, Di Mari L, Cianci A. Placebo-controlled study on efficacy and safety of daily apomorphine SL intake in premenopausal women affected by hypoactive sexual desire disorder and sexual arousal disorder. Urology. 2004;63:955–9. Annotation: A total of 50 women affected by arousal disorders and hypoactive sexual desire disorder participated. Daily apomorphine SL may improve the sexual life of women affected by sexual difficulties.

Ferguson DM, Steidle CP, Singh GS, Alexander JS, Weihmiller MK, Crosby MG. Randomized, placebo-controlled, double blind, crossover design trial of the efficacy and safety of Zestra for Women in women with and without female sexual arousal disorder. J Sex Marital Ther. 2003;29:S33-44. Annotation: This very small study of 10 women studied Zestra for Women as a botanical feminine massage oil formulated to enhance female sexual pleasure and arousal when applied to the vulva in home use. This over the counter product showed promise in improving sexual function.

Laan E, van Lunsen RH, Everaerd W, Riley A, Scott E, Boolell M. The enhancement of vaginal vasocongestion by sildenafil in healthy premenopausal women. J Womens Health Gend Based Med. 2002;11:357–65. Annotation: A total of 12 healthy pre-menopausal women without sexual dysfunction were randomly assigned to receive either a single oral 50 mg dose of sildenafil or matching placebo in a first session and the alternate medication in a second session. Significant increases in vaginal vasocongestion were found with sildenafil treatment compared with placebo during erotic stimulus conditions.

Nurnberg HG, Hensley PL, Gelenberg AJ, Fava M, Lauriello J, Paine S. Treatment of antidepressant-associated sexual dysfunction with sildenafil: a randomized controlled trial. JAMA. 2003;289:56–64. Annotation: A total of 90 men with sexual dysfunction associated with the use of selective and non-selective serotonin reuptake inhibitor anti-depressants participated. A total of 55% of sildenafil compared with 4% of placebo patients were much or very much improved. Sexual arousal, orgasm, and overall satisfaction domain measures improved significantly in sildenafil compared with placebo patients.

Sipski ML, Rosen RC, Alexander CJ, Hamer RM. Sildenafil effects on sexual and cardiovascular responses in women with spinal cord injury. Urology. 2000;55:812–5. Annotation: A total of 19 pre-menopausal women with spinal cord injuries were randomly assigned to receive either sildenafil or placebo in a double-blind, crossover design study. Significant increases in subjective arousal were observed with both drug and sexual stimulation conditions. Maximal responses occurred when sildenafil was combined with visual and manual sexual stimulation.

Vibrators and Devices

The EROS-Clitoral Therapy Device™ is the first FDA approved device for the treatment of women with sexual dysfunction. The clitoral vacuum device works by increasing blood flow to the clitoris and external genitalia. It is a small, handheld suction device, connected by tubing to a small, soft plastic cup that is placed over the clitoris. When a gentle vacuum is created, blood flow to the genitalia causes genital engorgement, increased vaginal lubrication, and enhanced ability to achieve orgasm. The EROS device may be used prior to having intercourse. Alternatively, the device may be used without intercourse, 3–4 times per week, to "rehabilitate" sexual responses.

If a woman is concerned that vaginal penetration will be uncomfortable, especially if her partner tends to get too enthusiastic, she may consider the use of a sexual aid, such as a vibrator, to prepare herself. Vaginal vibrators are made in the shape of a phallus, with or without a clitoral stimulator attached to the shaft. Bumps or ribs to help stimulate the vaginal erogenous zones more intensively cover some devices. Some are equipped with a separate control, with or without a wire. The devices usually have variable speeds, and may have vibrating motors that can be activated and controlled independently. A waterproof function allows use of a vibrator in or out of water. Multi-speed devices can be adjusted from slow to high for the intensity a woman wishes. Different women have different needs and respond individually to the sexual stimulation. However, for some women, vaginal penetration may simply be too painful.

Vibrators can be helpful in reducing pelvic floor muscle tension. If a woman has discomfort with a finger or tampon inside the vagina, this is more likely a consequence of pelvic floor muscle tension. Under such circumstances, physical therapy and muscle relaxation are the primary treatments. Vaginal penetration should *never* be forced. A vibrator may be used externally and/or internally to massage and relax the pelvic floor muscles. If possible, placement of a vaginal vibrator internally may enable one to specifically relax tender pelvic floor muscles.

If embarrassment is an issue, a woman can substitute a vaginal vibrator with a vibrator designed for other areas, such as her lower back, neck or feet. Such a vibrator can be placed directly on a woman's perineum or lower abdomen to help relax the pelvic floor muscles. If a woman has never used a vibrator before, the pelvic floor muscles commonly involved in painful penetration are located at the floor of the vagina and just to the side of the rectum. To massage those muscles, as the vibrator is entering, gently push the vibrator down towards the rectum and from side to side. When selecting the correct vibrator, size is important. A simple rule, especially if there is pain or discomfort, is that if the vibrator requires a double A battery, it may be the correct small size. If the vibrator requires a larger C or D battery, the vibrator may too wide.

Vibrators can be an enhancement to lovemaking and a source of personal pleasure. They are devices intended to vibrate against the body, including inside the vagina, thus stimulating the sensory nerves and enabling a pleasurable and possibly erotic feeling. Vibrators often allow women to achieve orgasm. A vibrator may stimulate vaginal sensory erogenous zones as well as the clitoris simultaneously, allowing a woman to experience pleasurable sensations. Vibrators may provide more intense orgasms than those produced by hand stimulation alone. These devices are often recommended by sex therapists for women who have difficulty reaching orgasm by other means. Vibrators may be used for self-stimulation purposes, or by a couple during mutual masturbation. Couples also use them to enhance the pleasure of one or both partners.

Lack of moisture may cause irritation and painful sensations when using a vibrator, therefore lubrication may be required. Many vibrators come with suitable lubricant because some substances can damage the texture of the vibrators. Vibrators can be pliable to create the feel of the real body and can be made out of silicone, jelly, rubber, vinyl or latex materials. Silicone retains body heat, has no odor, and warms up quickly. Silicone vibrators are easier to clean and care for since this material is not porous and bacteria do not remain on the surface. Silicone vibrators can be boiled up to 3 minutes or run through the dishwasher. In contrast, jelly material is porous and carries the scent of rubber. In order to mask this smell, some manufacturers aromatize the products with more pleasurable scents. Jelly materials cannot be sterilized in boiled water. For some polymer vibrators, it is preferable to replace them, as they are impossible to keep clean. Oil products, such as oil-based lubricants, massage oils, butter, and olive oil, can injure latex. Rubber vibrators are porous and often need more care to clean. They should always be used with condoms and cleaned with mild soap and water. Vinyl vibrators are light in weight, easy to clean, and come in many different forms and colors. Vinyl products are non-porous, and can be washed with mild soap and hot water.

References for Vibrators and Devices:

Billups KL, Berman L, Berman J, Metz ME, Glennon ME, Goldstein I. A new non-pharmacological vacuum therapy for female sexual dysfunction. J Sex Marital Ther. 2001;27:435–41. Annotation: The EROS-Clitoral Therapy Device™ is the first FDA cleared-to-market therapy for female sexual dysfunction. The EROS-Clitoral Therapy Device is a small, battery-powered device designed to increase clitoral blood flow, genital sensation, vaginal lubrication, ability to reach orgasm, and sexual satisfaction in women with female sexual dysfunction.

Billups KL. The role of mechanical devices in treating female sexual dysfunction and enhancing the female sexual response. World J Urol. 2002;20:137–41. Annotation: Mechanical devices may cause clitoral vascular engorgement using a vacuum system. The EROS device is a small, battery-powered device used to gently apply direct vacuum over the clitoris causing the clitoral erectile chambers and labia to fill with blood.

Leiblum SR. Arousal disorders in women: complaints and complexities. Med J Aust. 2003;178:638–40. Annotation: Female sexual arousal disorders constitute a varied spectrum of difficulties. The most common complaint is the absence of subjective sexual excitement or pleasure despite adequate physical arousal (e.g., lubrication). Physical treatments include the use of lubricants and vibrators. Psychological therapy addresses inhibitions, and interpersonal and motivational factors.

Meston CM, Hull E, Levin RJ, Sipski M. Disorders of orgasm in women. J Sex Med. 2004;1:66–8. Annotation: Orgasm is a sensation of intense pleasure creating an altered consciousness state accompanied by pelvic striated circumvaginal musculature and uterine/anal contractions and myotonia resolving sexually induced vasocongestion and inducing wellbeing/contentment. Empirical treatment outcome research is available for cognitive behavioral approaches. Cognitive-behavioral therapy for anorgasmia uses behavioral exercises including directed masturbation.

Schroder M, Mell LK, Hurteau JA, Collins YC, Rotmensch J, Waggoner SE, Yamada SD, Small W Jr, Mundt AJ. Clitoral therapy device for treatment of sexual dysfunction in irradiated cervical cancer patients. Int J Radiat Oncol Biol Phys. 2005;61:1078–86. Annotation: A total of 13 women with a history of cervical cancer were treated with radiotherapy. They reported symptoms of sexual arousal and/or orgasmic disorders; some also had sexual desire and pain disorders. Patients used the clitoral therapy device for clitoral engorgement 4 times weekly for 3 months during foreplay and self-stimulation. At 3 months, statistically significant improvements were seen in all domains tested, including sexual desire, arousal, lubrication, orgasm, sexual satisfaction, and reduced pain.

Gynecologic examinations revealed improved mucosal color and moisture and vaginal elasticity, as well as decreased bleeding and ulceration.

Segraves RT. Emerging therapies for female sexual dysfunction. Expert Opin Emerg Drugs. 2003;8:515–22. Annotation: Epidemiological studies in the US, the UK, and Sweden indicate that approximately 40% of women aged 18–59 have significant complaints about their sexual lives. A common problem is difficulty reaching orgasm. A vacuum clitoris therapy device that increases blood flow to the clitoris has been approved by the US Food and Drug Administration.

Physical Therapy for Female Sexual Dysfunction

Talli Yehuda Rosenbaum, B.S., P.T.

Urogynecological Physiotherapist
AASECT Certified Sexual Counselor
Bet Shemesh, Israel

Physical Therapy

Professionals involved in sexual health have traditionally included educators, counselors, therapists, and physicians, particularly in specialties such as psychiatry, gynecology, and urology. The inclusion of physical therapists in the team of professionals involved in promoting sexual health and in treating sexual dysfunction is a relatively recent advancement. Physical therapists are trained to provide treatment to restore function, improve mobility, relieve pain, and prevent or limit permanent physical disabilities of patients suffering from injuries or disease. As community health professionals, physical therapists are involved in health and fitness education and promoting wellness. As sexual health is an integral component to overall wellness, and sexual activity a valued human activity, physical therapists in various settings have an important role in promoting sexual health and treating dysfunction.

Within physical therapy is a specialty known as urogynecological rehabilitation. Physical therapists involved in this specialty are trained in the treatment of disorders related to the pelvic floor. Pelvic floor disorders include urinary dysfunction such as incontinence (unwanted loss of urine) urgency, and frequency, as well as organ prolapse, which refers to a situation where the bladder, uterus, and/or rectum "fall" downwards into the vaginal canal. Pelvic floor disorders due to muscle weakness contribute to these conditions and sexual dysfunction has been found to be closely associated with them. Low libido, vaginal dryness, painful intercourse, decreased orgasm rates and intensity, and decreased overall sexual satisfaction have been reported in women with urinary incontinence. The relationship between urological and sexual problems has prompted the suggestion that women with urinary problems be questioned about their sexual function. The literature does support the use of pelvic floor strengthening exercises with physical therapy to improve quality of life and sexual function in women with urinary stress incontinence.

The physical therapist is an important member of the team of professionals treating sexual pain disorders. Pelvic floor hypertonus (high muscle tone) dysfunction is a component of sexual pain, and an important part of physical therapy is teaching the patient how to normalize muscle tone. The physical therapy intervention generally consists of evaluation and treatment with education and cognitive behavioral therapy, exercises, manual therapy techniques, and modalities including pelvic floor biofeedback and electrical stimulation.

The physical therapy approach to the treatment of women with complaints of inability to have intercourse, or painful intercourse, includes taking a detailed history, performing a physical exam, and providing a treatment plan together with the patient. Physical therapists provide education, anatomical and physiological information, and give specific exercises with the goals of decreasing pain with intercourse and allowing vaginal penetration mobility. Physical therapists provide exercises to decrease the sensitivity of the painful tissues. Manual techniques, including massage, stretching, soft tissue and bony mobilizations, are important components of treatment. Patients are often taught how to use gradual vaginal dilators to overcome the anxiety involved in penetration as well as to help stretch the vaginal tissue. Pelvic floor sEMG (surface electromyography) biofeedback is one of the many tools available and commonly used by physical therapists in the treatment of vulvar pain syndromes. In EMG biofeedback, a sensor is placed in the vagina and the muscle activity of the pelvic floor is recorded and displayed on a computer monitor. With this visual feedback, the woman is able to see how tense or weak her muscles are, and this allows her to learn the proper methods to relax and strengthen her muscles.

References for Physical Therapy:

Bo K, Talseth T, Vinsnes A. Randomized controlled trial on the effect of pelvic floor muscle training on quality of life and sexual problems in genuine stress incontinent women. Acta Obstet Gynecol Scand. 2000;79:598–603. Annotation: This is an important trial that demonstrates that pelvic floor exercises are effective in curing urinary stress incontinence in women.

Handa VL, Harvey L, Cundiff GW, Kjerulff KH. Sexual function among women with urinary incontinence and pelvic organ prolapse. Am J Obstet Gynecol. 2004;191:751–6. Annotation: This study of 1299 women concludes that women with disorders of the pelvic floor, particularly stress incontinence, have a higher likelihood of experiencing sexual problems than women without pelvic floor problems.

Pauls, RN, Berman JR. Impact of pelvic floor disorders and prolapse of female sexual function and response. Urol Clin North Am. 2002;29:677–83. Annotation: Pelvic floor problems are likely to affect women's sexual wellbeing through physical and emotional effects. Women with pelvic floor disorders often have co-existing urologic and sexual complaints. Patients who present with these urologic problems should be questioned about their sexual function.

Rosenbaum T. Physiotherapy treatment of sexual pain disorders. J Sex Marital Ther. 2005;31:329–40. Annotation: This article describes how physiotherapy can be utilized in treating sexual pain disorders.

Sex Therapy for Female Sexual Dysfunction

Sandra Leiblum, Ph.D.

Director, Center for Sexual and Relationship Health
Robert Wood Johnson Medical School
Piscataway, New Jersey

Sex Therapy

Sex therapy provides a forum where all of the contributions to sexual difficulties can be identified and addressed, with the woman alone and with her partner, if she has one. In most instances, therapy begins with a careful and systematic assessment of the factors contributing to the current difficulty. What were the attitudes of the woman's family towards nudity, affection, open discussion of sexuality, pre-marital sex? What positive or negative experiences did she have in her close or intimate relationships growing up, both sexual and non-sexual? When and how did she meet her primary partner? How attracted was she initially? How attracted is she currently? Does she feel safe, cared for, valued, and respected, both in and out of bed? Are the environmental conditions conducive to sexual abandonment? Is she worried about the children, her in-laws or distracted by the thought of others in the house? Is the room warm or cool enough? Does she feel physically attractive? Does she feel sexually receptive, even if she does not feel intrinsic sexual interest, or does she feel obligated to engage in sex in order to avoid alienating or angering her spouse? Is she generally satisfied with the emotional intimacy she has with her partner, or does she feel resentful, detached or angry? Is there adequate stimulation (in the right places and for long enough periods of time) to facilitate mental and genital arousal and sexual desire? These are just a few of the kinds of questions that are explored during the initial assessment and throughout sex therapy.

A comprehensive medical review of systems is undertaken as well, including hormonal assessment (in cases where estrogen or androgen deficiency is suspected). The therapist asks about past surgeries and acute or chronic illness as well as current use of both prescription and over the counter medications. A thorough assessment should include questions about the woman and her partner's ethnic or cultural background, religious devoutness, sexual beliefs and expectations, and goals of therapy, e.g., procreation? pleasure? Further, the therapist wants to learn as much as possible about the woman's past enjoyment and satisfaction with sensual or sexual activities, typical sexual response, and comfort with sexual behaviors, including oral-genital sex, fantasy or use of erotic media.

If a woman has never enjoyed sex, treatment may be challenging. However, if a woman can recall past pleasurable sexual feelings or experiences and past or present loving relationships, the prognosis is usually quite good. It is often possible to rekindle sexual desire and/or resolve sexual problems psychotherapeutically if a woman has experienced and enjoyed sexual intimacy and relationship fulfillment with a current partner and wants to recapture it, rather than if she is trying to comply with an irate partner's demands for more or frequent sex.

While sexual apathy or diminished sexual desire is the most prevalent sexual complaint of women, orgasmic problems are common as well. In general, women with orgasm difficulties tend to experience more sexual guilt, are less sexually assertive, and endorse more negative attitudes towards sexual activity and masturbation than do orgasmic women. Many orgasmic women fear loss of control with orgasm and this, along with other fears or misconceptions, can be identified and discussed in sex therapy treatment.

Directed masturbation training has been found to be the most effective psychologic treatment for lifelong and generalized orgasmic problems, and education and permission to engage in self-stimulation may be the first (and often, most effective) intervention for the woman who has never experienced an orgasm. On the other hand, women with acquired and situational orgasmic problems tend to be less satisfied with their overall relationship than women with primary orgasmic dysfunction, so that sex therapy may focus on couples' treatment and resolution of on-going relationship dissatisfactions. Most psychologic treatment approaches for orgasmic difficulties include a combination of sex education, sexual skills training, couple's therapy, masturbation, and non-demand touching exercises, as well as interventions to address body image concerns and negative sexual attitudes.

Women often come to sex therapy complaining of a variety of sexual pain complaints. In such instances, a careful medical evaluation is recommended to determine whether there are structural or anatomical issues, nerve damage, infections, lesions, hormonal insufficiencies, etc. that may be either responsible for, or contributing to the problem. Vulvodynia or vulvar vestibulitis is a fairly common problem in women and is often best treated by a multidisciplinary team of specialists, including gynecologists, psychologists, sexual medicine physicians, physical therapists etc. Medications, massage, and non-demand sensual exercises can all be helpful in reducing sexual discomfort, and sex therapy to challenge the negative and worrisome thoughts that often accompany sexual pain problems is useful.

In conclusion, sex therapy can be very effective in helping women of all ages overcome and discover or return to a more satisfying sexual life. The well-trained sex therapist is someone who, in addition to good overall clinical skills in resolving anxiety and depression, fears and inhibitions, is skilled in working with couples and in treating sexual dissatisfactions and sexual dysfunctions. Therapy is typically brief, often no more than 10-12 sessions, but focused. Cognitive-behavioral interventions, permission and education, "homework" assignments, including suggestion for at-home sensual exercises or self-exploration, comprise some of the therapeutic options practiced by sex therapists. If the woman (and her partner) is motivated to achieve a more satisfying, lasting sexual and intimate relationship, sex therapy is the treatment of choice.

References for Sex Therapy:

Althof S, Leiblum S, Chevret-Measson M, Hartmann U, Levine S, McCabe M. Plaut M, Rodriques O, Wylie K. Psychological and Interpersonal Contributions to Male and Female Sexual Dysfunction. J Sex Med. 2005;2:793–800. Annotation: Comprehensive evidence-based review of psychological factors that contribute to sexual dysfunction.

Binik Y, Bergeron S, Khalife S. Dyspareunia and Vaginismus: So called sexual pain. In: Leiblum SR, ed. Principles and practice of sex therapy, 4th ed. Guilford Press: New York, 2007. Annotation: Review of sexual pain disorders and recommendations for an interdisciplinary treatment approach to the relief of sexual pain.

Heiman J. (2007). Orgasmic Disorders in Women. In: Leiblum SR, ed. Principles and practice of sex therapy, 4th ed. Guilford Press: New York, 2007. Annotation: A comprehensive review of etiological, maintaining, and treatment approaches to orgasmic complaints in women.

Leiblum S, Wiegel M. Psychotherapeutic interventions for treating female sexual dysfunction. World J Urol. 2002;20:127–36. Annotation: A review of cognitive behavioral treatments for womens' sexual dysfunctions, including descriptions of each of the various interventions.

Afterword

We have interviewed many women in the course of writing this book. Based on our discussions with them, it became clear to us that there was a paucity of information available to them about women's sexual health. For that reason, we have chosen to devote half of this book to the science of sexual medicine, written in a manner that we hope is clear and comprehensible. Armed with this knowledge, women have a better opportunity to be attentive to their sexual health. They no longer need to accept the statement that sexual problems are, "all in your head."

This unique combination of stories and science as well as the extensive reference material has been written and designed especially for our readers. We hope you have found it to be helpful. We also hope that you will feel comfortable bringing this book with you when discussing your sexual health with your healthcare provider.

About the Authors

Lillian Arleque is a nationally known motivational speaker, educator, and consultant. Providing trail-blazing and humorous keynote addresses, seminars, and workshops for business, academia, and the medical community, Dr. Arleque leaves her "pioneering spirit" on the lives of her audience participants. In addition to speaking, Dr. Arleque is a leadership coach, helping men and women regain control of their professional lives, author of a chapter in *Women's Sexual Function and Dysfunction*, the first textbook on women's sexual health, and a member of the International Society for the Study of Women's Sexual Health.

Dr. Arleque earned her doctorate in education from the University of Massachusetts. She has had more than twenty-four years of teaching experience and fifteen years of speaking experience, and more recently has co-chaired and been a speaker at sexual medicine education seminars. Dr. Goldstein has used Dr. Arleque as a patient resource on numerous occasions. Dr. Arleque decided to take her knowledge to the next level by co-authoring her first book. In this way, she is fulfilling her dream, as well as providing a valuable service.

Sue W. Goldstein worked in an endocrinology laboratory after graduating from Brown University. After taking time off to raise her children, she reentered the work force in her first love, education. After several years working as a technical writer in the field of sexual medicine, Ms. Goldstein was named coordinator of education and development for sexual medicine at a local medical school, responsible for organizing and funding educational programs for physicians in training, physicians in practice and the general public, including co-chairing several sexual medicine seminars with Dr. Arleque. Ms. Goldstein continues in this capacity in her new position at Alvarado Hospital.

Ms. Goldstein is also editorial assistant for *The Journal of Sexual Medicine*. She is Online Services Chair for the International Society for the Study of Women's Sexual Health, and an honorary member of the International Society for Sexual Medicine. In addition to authoring a chapter in *Women's Sexual Function and Dysfunction*, Ms. Goldstein served as an associate editor of this textbook that recently received an award of Highly Commended by the Royal Society of Medicine.

Both authors bring not only their professional expertise to this book, but their personal experiences of living with and managing their own sexual health issues.

Reference Section

Glossary of Terms

Androgens: Seven androgen or androgen precursor sex steroids. They share a similar structure in that they are 19 carbon sex steroids. Androgens and androgen precursors are produced primarily by the ovaries and adrenal glands, but also from other organs, such as skin, bone, and muscle. Four androgens can be routinely measured: dehydroepiandrosterone-sulfate; androstenedione; testosterone; and dihydrotestosterone. Androgens induce genital and non-genital cells to synthesize specific proteins, such as growth factors and enzymes. These proteins affect genital tissue growth, maintain genital tissue structure, and play a critical role in genital tissue physiology, including engorgement and blood flow changes with sexual stimulation. Androgen-induced proteins also affect sexual desire, bone density, adipose tissue (fat) distribution, mood, energy, and wellbeing. In many cases, lack of androgens can be associated with genital atrophy and sexual health problems. *See Medical Therapy Science Section/Androgen Therapy*

Androgen Insufficiency Syndrome: Pattern of clinical symptoms in the presence of low androgen blood test values. The clinical symptoms include decreased sexual interest, decreased energy, fatigue, and depression. The low androgen blood test values are best measured by "unbound" testosterone or "calculated free testosterone." The syndrome can be defined only when estrogen blood levels are normal.

Androgen Therapy: Systemic hormone treatment for women with sexual health issues, who are suspected to have androgen insufficiency syndrome and low levels of "unbound" or "calculated free testosterone." Androgen therapy may include dehydroepiandrosterone treatment and/or testosterone treatment. Testosterone treatment is approved in Europe for women with low sexual desire and surgical menopause. Testosterone treatment is not yet approved in the United States for women with sexual health concerns, and thus its use is considered "off-label." Ideally, the dose of androgens delivered daily to women with sexual health concerns is designed to keep the blood levels of the various androgens in the mid to upper values of the normal range. Blood levels for dehydroepiandrosterone and testosterone are typically checked every 3 months while on therapy, until stable values are achieved.

Data show that women with sexual health concerns, who have androgen insufficiency, have significantly improved sexual function using androgen therapy. Potential adverse effects of androgen (dehydroepiandrosterone and/or testosterone) therapy include facial hair growth (hirsutism) and acne. There is no evidence that exogenous testosterone increases the risk of endometrial cancer, endometriosis, breast cancer, cardiovascular concerns, sleep apnea or aggressiveness. Issues such as balding, voice deepening, and enlarged clitoris do not result when dosing used for women with sexual health problems is selected as 10% of the usual male dose for hypogonadism. *See Medical Therapy Science Section/Androgen Therapy*

Aromatase: Enzyme that facilitates the conversion of testosterone to estradiol, and androstenedione to estrone. Having an active aromatase enzyme allows women to be treated with testosterone for low testosterone values and receive the benefit of diminished intensity of hot flashes and night sweats (an estrogen effect). As women age, the activity of the aromatase enzyme appears to diminish, so that testosterone conversion to estradiol is reduced. *See Medical Therapy Science Section/Androgen Therapy*

Arousal: Feelings and physical signs of sexual desire. Arousal may be sub-classified into 3 specific categories: subjective, genital, and combined. Subjective sexual arousal consists of feelings of sexual arousal, sexual excitement, and sexual pleasure derived from any type of sexual stimulation. It does not always strongly correlate with genital congestion. Genital sexual arousal consists of vulvar swelling or vaginal lubrication from any type of sexual stimulation, and sexual sensations from caressing genitalia. Combined genital and subjective arousal includes feelings of sexual arousal, sexual excitement, and sexual pleasure from any type of sexual stimulation, as well as genital sexual arousal, such as vulvar swelling or vaginal lubrication.

Atrophy: Shrinking in size of some part or organ of the body, usually caused by lack of hormone (androgens or estrogens) support, injury, aging or reduced blood flow.

Bartholin's Glands: Situated at the bottom of the posterior parts of the labia minora, deep to the lowest inner portions of the clitoris (crus), and deep to the erectile tissue of the corpora spongiosa. The right and left greater (major) vestibular glands produce a clear, mucinous secretion during sexual arousal, designed to aid in physiologic vestibular lubrication. The main duct of each Bartholin's gland opens at the side of the lower half of the vaginal opening, near the hymen. The Bartholin's glands may be the site of infection and cyst formation. *See Illustrations*

Bioavailable Testosterone: Records the sum of the "unbound" testosterone, as well as the loosely bound testosterone, to albumin. Sex steroid hormones, such as testosterone, may be tightly "bound" to sex hormone binding globulin, loosely bound to albumin, or "unbound" to either protein, and physiologically available to enter the cell and direct protein synthesis. Bioavailable testosterone is considered more clinically useful than total testosterone, especially if sex hormone binding globulin values are elevated. *See Medical Therapy Science Section/Androgen Therapy*

Bioidentical Hormones: Made commercially to be chemically exact duplicates of the hormones and their precursors (7 androgens, 3 estrogens, and 1 progesterone) produced by the woman in her own body. One major reason why healthcare providers prefer bioidentical hormones for hormone therapy is that they can be measured scientifically and accurately with standard blood testing. Bioidentical hormones can be extracted and derived from a variety of different sources, e.g., soy or yams. Bioidentical hormones, such as testosterone, estradiol, and progesterone, can be obtained as FDA-approved products in traditional pharmacies. FDA-approved products are recommended, especially since the important drug manufacturing process is carefully inspected by the FDA. Bioidentical hormones can also be obtained as non-FDA-approved products in compounding pharmacies. The manufacturing process of compounded products is not inspected by the FDA, and concentrations of the hormones may vary within the solution (layering effect within the ointment or cream) or may vary from one compounding pharmacist to another.

Biofeedback: Use of a monitoring device that displays information about the operation of a bodily function that is not normally consciously controlled, such as heart rate or body temperature. Electromyographic (EMG) biofeedback monitors muscle activity, which is under conscious control. Electromyography provides the woman with visual and auditory feedback to relax and strengthen the pelvic floor muscles. *See Physical Therapy Science Section*

Breast Cancer Susceptibility Gene (BRCA): Breast cancer receptor gene that shows increased risk of breast and ovarian cancer. The changes from normal in the $BRCA_1$ or $BRCA_2$ genes can be inherited from your mother or father.

Genetic counseling is imperative, as having the BRCA gene does not mean you have cancer.

C-Reactive Protein: Blood test that measures the concentration of a protein that indicates new inflammation. Recent studies have suggested that inflammation is important in the process in which fatty deposits build up in the lining of arteries, or atherosclerosis. C-reactive protein levels, using the very high sensitivity assay called "hs-CRP," may assess for cardiovascular disease risk. Researchers are finding that hs-CRP levels can predict recurrent cardiovascular disease, stroke, and death. If the hs-CRP level is lower than 1.0 mg/L, a person has a low risk of developing cardiovascular disease. If hs-CRP is between 1.0 and 3.0 mg/L, a person has an average risk. If hs-CRP is higher than 3.0 mg/L, a person is at high risk.

Since blood flow is an important biologic aspect of sexual arousal, it is important to note elevated C-reactive protein levels that may predict individuals with impaired blood flow and sexual dysfunction. Using this hypothesis, C-reactive protein levels were measured in women at risk for blood vessel inflammation, that is, women with metabolic syndrome. Compared to women without metabolic syndrome, it has been found that women with metabolic syndrome have lower sexual function scores, lower sexual satisfaction, and higher levels of C-reactive protein. Strategies to lower elevated C-reactive protein levels include diet, exercise, and statins (drugs that are very effective in reducing cholesterol). *See Medical Therapy Science Section/Mediterranean Diet*

Clitoris: Erectile structure approximately five inches (thirteen centimeters) in length, of which only a small segment, the glans clitoris, is noticeable from the vestibule surface. The shaft or body of the clitoris is comprised of two paired erectile chambers passing upwards underneath the vulva, towards the pubic bone, and continuing as separate right and left clitoral curae, straddling the urethra and vagina. During sexual arousal, clitoral blood flow increases and clitoral smooth muscle relaxes. The result is that the engorged portion of the clitoris not attached to the pelvic bone, the clitoris shaft, changes its angle to the vulva from thirty degrees at baseline to more than ninety degrees during sexual arousal. The increased angle improves opportunity for clitoral glans contact during sexual activity. *See Illustrations*

Dehydroepiandrosterone (DHEA): Androgen precursor in a woman's body that ultimately converts to testosterone. Dehydroepiandrosterone is the first of the androgen precursors, synthesized primarily in the adrenal gland. Dehydroepiandrosterone treatment has been shown to improve sexual desire, arousal, lubrication, orgasm, and satisfaction in women with sexual dysfunction. Dehydroepiandrosterone has multiple actions including helping arterial blood vessels relax. There are no FDA-approved dehydroepiandrosterone products, however, bioidentical dehydroepiandrosterone is commonly purchased at health food stores. *See Medical Therapy Science Section/Androgen Therapy*

Dopamine: Appears to play a role in central sexual arousal, sexual excitation, sexual mood, and sexual motivation. In animal research, dopamine neurotransmitter systems may promote the craving or desire for continued sexual activity once sexual stimulation has started. Treatment with dopaminergic agonist drugs (agents that act like dopamine) has resulted in an increase in sexual desire and improvement in orgasm in a number of women with sexual dysfunction.

Dyspareunia: A sexual pain disorder, defined as a recurrent and persistent genital pain, experienced in varying genital locations. Pre-menopausal dyspareunia can be secondary to vulvar vestibulitis syndrome, vestibular dermatologic conditions such as lichen sclerosis or lichen planus, or fungal infections of the clitoris or labia. Deep dyspareunia is associated with pelvic pathology such as endometriosis and chronic pelvic pain, associated with pelvic floor disorders. Other causes of dyspareunia include Bartholin cysts, fibroepitheliomas of the frenulum, interstitial cystitis, and sexually transmitted diseases such as herpes or human papilomavirus. Post-menopausal dyspareunia is commonly due to vaginal atrophy and reduced lubrication, secondary to low estradiol blood levels. Genital pain is a multi-dimensional physical and psychologic health concern. *See Medical Factors Science Section/Vulvodynia*

EMEA: European Medicines Agency, a regulatory body for pharmaceutical and device products in the European Union.

Endometriosis: Condition where endometrium uterine lining tissue is found growing outside the uterus. The endometrial tissue, even when outside the uterus, responds to hormone alterations during the menstrual cycle. The most common symptoms of endometriosis are painful menstrual periods and/or pelvic pain. Endometriosis is a cause of sexual pain or dyspareunia affecting 10% to 15% of pre-menopausal women.

Endothelium: Innermost lining of the blood vessels. The endothelium plays a critical role in the health of the blood vessel. The endothelium is instrumental in communicating to the adjacent blood vessel muscular layer to regulate blood vessel dilation or contraction. The endothelium also plays a central role in blood vessel inflammation. A healthy endothelium provides a protective coating. When endothelium is damaged, inflammation occurs, leading to atherosclerosis or fatty deposits narrowing the lumen of the blood vessel. Nitric oxide is synthesized in endothelial cells, diffusing freely across cell membranes into smooth muscle cells causing them to relax, and assisting blood flow through the vessels. Nitric oxide inhibits blood vessel inflammation.

Estrogens: Three estrogen sex steroids: estrone, estradiol, and estriol. They share a similar structure in that they are 18 carbon sex steroids. The most clinically important is estradiol, synthesized from androgens via the enzyme aromatase. Estrogens induce genital and non-genital cells to synthesize specific proteins, such as growth factors and enzymes. These proteins affect genital tissue growth, maintain genital tissue structure, and play a critical role in genital tissue physiology, including engorgement and blood flow changes with sexual stimulation. Estrogen-induced proteins also affect the development, growth, and maintenance of many organs and tissues in women, including the mammary gland, genital tissue, bone, and skin. In many cases, lack of estrogens can be associated with genital atrophy and sexual health problems, such as decreased pelvic blood flow, diminished vaginal lubrication, and thinning of the vaginal wall. *See Medical Therapy Science Section/Estrogen Therapy*

Estrogen Therapy: Systemic (affecting the whole body) or local (directed only to the vagina or vestibule) treatment indicated in women with sexual health concerns that may be related to low estradiol and symptoms of estrogen insufficiency. At menopause, estradiol concentrations in the blood fall to low levels. This decrease is often accompanied by estrogen insufficiency symptoms such as vascular instability (hot flashes and night sweats), changes in mood and concentration, sleep disturbances, fatigue and diminished energy, a rise in the incidence of heart disease, and an increasing rate of bone loss (osteoporosis). There is growing evidence that alterations in the estradiol blood levels may contribute to sexual health problems. Adequate estrogen levels are important in preserving genital tissue structure and function and, in particular, to vestibular and vaginal sexual receptiveness. Estrogen insufficiency symptoms may include complaints about sexual desire, arousal, lubrication, orgasm, and sexual pain.
There is no one estrogen intervention (systemic, local or a combination of both) that will be effective for all women with sexual health concerns caused, in part, by low levels of estrogen and/or estrogen insufficiency. Systemic and local estradiol treatments have been shown to re-establish vaginal integrity and lubrication in post-menopausal women with low levels of estradiol. Systemic

therapy, in particular, increases pelvic blood flow and improves sexual desire, arousal, orgasm, and frequency of sexual activity.

Among the most common estrogen side effects are break-through bleeding or spotting, excessively prolonged periods, breast pain, and breast enlargement. Migraine headaches and sodium and fluid retention have been associated with estrogen therapy. Cigarette smokers are at a higher risk for blood clots, therefore, patients requiring estrogen therapy are strongly encouraged not to smoke. Estrogens can promote a buildup of the uterine lining and endometrial hyperplasia, and increase the risk of endometrial carcinoma. The addition of a progestin to estrogen therapy helps prevent endometrial carcinoma. There may be a small increase in risk of breast cancer. *See Medical Therapy Science Section/ Estrogen Therapy*

Estrogen Therapy (Local): Can successfully improve local symptoms such as vaginal lubrication, dryness, and dyspareunia. Local vaginal or vestibular estrogen therapy has no effect on systemic estrogen insufficiency symptoms, such as night sweats and hot flashes. Local vaginal or vestibular estrogen therapy improves vaginal or vestibular health, including improved tissue perfusion, lubrication, tissue tone, and elasticity. Local vaginal estrogen therapy restores normal acidic vaginal pH. Some systemic absorption occurs with local estrogen delivery, especially for the first few weeks of local vaginal estrogen therapy, if the woman's vaginal lining is very thin. Studies have shown that local vaginal estradiol treatments can be used with caution in women with breast cancer. One study in women with breast cancer showed that local vaginal estrogen use was not associated with an increase in the breast cancer recurrence rate.

Estrogen Therapy (Systemic): Can successfully improve both local (genital atrophy, genital pain) and systemic (hot flashes, night sweats, and sleep disturbances) symptoms of estrogen insufficiency that negatively affect body image, mood, and sexual desire. During estrogen therapy, one strategy is to maintain estradiol values at low levels (approximately 50 pg/ml) to reduce side effects (breast cancer, heart attack, and stroke) and to achieve efficacy treating estrogen insufficiency symptoms. In women with an intact uterus, systemic estrogen should always be opposed by a progestin.

FDA: Food and Drug Administration, a regulatory body in the United States for pharmaceutical and device products.

Female Androgen Insufficiency Syndrome: See Androgen Insufficiency Syndrome

Female Prostate (Skene's Glands): Empties through ejaculatory ducts. The duct openings often exit on either side of the urethral meatus but can exit in varying locations, including the urethra and between the labia and hymenal tissue. During orgasm, the female prostate expresses fluid that contains prostate specific antigen and prostate specific acid phosphatase, not urine. *See Illustrations*

Female Sexual Dysfunction (FSD): Psychological and physiological persistent or recurrent disorder of desire, arousal, orgasm, and/or pain causing personal distress.

Female Sexual Function Index (FSFI): Widely used self-report questionnaire that has been extensively validated in numerous clinical trials of women with female sexual arousal disorder (FASD), hypoactive sexual desire disorder (HSDD), sexual pain disorders, and multiple sexual dysfunctions. The FSFI consists of 19 items that assess women's sexual feelings and responses in the areas of sexual desire, subjective sexual arousal, lubrication, orgasm, satisfaction with sexual activity, and pain.

Fibroids: Benign growth in the wall of the uterus composed of fibrous and muscle tissue, often associated with painful cramps and excessive menstrual flow.

Free Testosterone Level: Free or "unbound" testosterone values measured by a blood test called "analog free testosterone." This test, however, is not reliable. "Unbound" testosterone is better assessed employing an online tool to determine "calculated free testosterone," utilizing the blood value results for albumin, total testosterone, and sex hormone binding globulin. "Calculated free testosterone" is one of the best ways to determine whether a woman has sufficient "unbound" testosterone for her physiologic needs. *See Medical Therapy Science Section/Androgen Therapy*

Frenulum: Highly sensitive tissues that emanate to the left and right off the lower aspect of the glans clitoris. The right and left frenulae continue to form the right and left labia minora. The frenulae may be among the most sensitive locations of the woman's genital area. *See Illustrations*

G-spot (Grafenberg Spot): Sexually sensitive area in the upper vaginal wall, near the junction of the bladder and the urethra. The G-spot is not a spot but a gland, the female prostate, also called Skene's gland. During ejaculation, the female prostate tissue releases fluid containing the same protein, prostate specific antigen, in women as in men. *See Illustrations*

Genital Herpes: Sexually transmitted disease caused by the herpes simplex virus, affecting the genital and anal regions, associated with painful lesions. Sexually transmitted diseases adversely affect sexual function by causing pain and by decreasing sexual interest and arousal.

Genitalia (External): Includes all the structures surrounding the vulva. The anatomy of the surface of the external genitalia differs noticeably among women. In some, the surface anatomy includes only the mons and labia majora. Unless the labia are parted, the labia minora and clitoris may not be seen. *See Illustrations*

Genitalia (Internal): All the structures of the vestibule, including the clitoris, the prepuce (hood) of the clitoris, the right and left frenulum, the urethral opening (meatus), the labia minora, the ducts of the major (Bartholin) and minor vestibular glands, the hymen, the vaginal opening, and all the nerves, arteries, and veins to the skin surface in the region. *See Illustrations*

Genital Sensation Test: Test to assess the sensation of the genital skin, especially the clitoris, labia minora, and urethral meatus, conducted in the physician's office. The test can measure skin vibration sensitivity with a device called a BioThesiometer™ or temperature sensitivity with a GenitoSensory Analyzer™. The woman is asked to inform the healthcare professional when she feels or does not feel the stimulus (vibration perception or temperature perception) on the tested area.

Genital Sexual Arousal: Response resulting in increased genital blood flow and relaxation of genital smooth muscle associated with sexual stimulation. Genital sexual arousal leads to physiologic changes to the clitoris, labia minora and corpora spongiosa, Bartholin's and minor vestibular glands, female prostate (G-spot, Skene's glands or periurethral ducts), and vagina. During genital sexual arousal, there is increased length and width of the clitoris, and increased angle of the shaft and glans clitoris to the vestibule. There is increased width of the corpora spongiosa surrounding the vaginal opening helping to keep the erect penis inside the vagina. There is gland lubrication from the Bartholin's and minor vestibular glands to aid in painless penetration. There is lengthening and widening of the vagina, increased vaginal lubrication, and increased production of lubricating mucus from the cervix. These physiological events are dependent upon the health of the genital tissues and the function of neural, endocrine, and vascular systems that regulate and coordinate the genital sexual arousal response.

Hood (of the Clitoris): Fold of tissue (prepuce) that partially or fully covers and protects the unstimulated clitoris. During sexual arousal, the glans clitoris protrudes from the clitoral hood. The hood can undergo atrophy if the woman has hormone insufficiency. The hood can become scarred and not allow the glans to protrude during sexual arousal. This is called phimosis of the clitoral prepuce. If pain or infection occurs on the glans clitoris because of phimosis (closed compartment syndrome), a surgical procedure, dorsal slit of the clitoral prepuce, can be performed under either local or regional anesthesia. There is no evidence that dorsal slit prepucial surgery improves orgasm in women without pain or infection of the prepuce. *See Illustrations*

Hormone: Chemical substance (e.g., estradiol) produced in the body's endocrine glands (e.g., ovary) that exerts a regulatory or stimulatory effect on another distant gland or tissue (e.g., breast). Hormones act by stimulating the hormonally sensitive cell to synthesize proteins, such as growth factors and enzymes.

Hot Flash (Hot Flush): Sudden feeling of heat in the upper part or all of the body, associated with face and neck flushing, and red blotches on the chest, back, and arms. Heavy sweating and cold shivering can follow. Hot flashes can be a light blush or night sweats severe enough to awaken a woman from a sound sleep, and can last from 30 seconds to 10 minutes. Hot flashes may be experienced during menopause and for several years after. They are caused by an endocrine imbalance and commonly treated by administration of systemic estradiol. Some women may be successfully treated by systemic androgens, since androgens convert to estrogens by the enzyme aromatase. Other treatments for hot flashes include selective serotonin reuptake inhibitors, although they have many sexual side effects. *See Medical Factors Science Section/Menopause*

Hymen: Thin, incomplete membrane of connective tissue at the junction of the vestibule and the vagina that varies widely in appearance. The hymen represents the junction of the inner vagina (80% of the total vagina) with the outer vagina (20% of the total vagina). The hymen may or may not rupture with intercourse or may rupture in certain physical activities unrelated to sex. After hymenal rupture, the hymen becomes small, round, fleshy tissue outgrowths just on the inside of the vaginal opening. Regular use of tampons, regular sexual intercourse or injury from childbirth will reduce the hymen to a series of irregular tissue thickenings around the vaginal opening. *See Illustrations*

Hypoactive Sexual Desire Disorder (HSDD): Persistent or recurrent deficiency and/or absence of sexual fantasies/thoughts, and/or desire for, or receptivity to, sexual activity that causes personal distress.

Hypogonadism: Having a physiologic "unbound" testosterone concentration below the normal range for healthy women. Values of "unbound" testosterone in the lowest quarter of the normal range are also considered suspicious for hypogonadism in a woman with sexual dysfunction. This is because the "normal" range was often determined including women with sexual dysfunction who were otherwise healthy. *See Medical Science Section/Androgen Therapy*

Hypothyroidism: Occurs when the thyroid does not produce sufficient thyroid hormone. Thyroid hormones are important and act to maintain fat and carbohydrate metabolism, control body temperature, and regulate protein production. Signs and symptoms of low thyroid hormone are varied and include: increased sensitivity to cold, constipation, pale and dry skin, unexplained weight gain, muscle aches, tenderness and stiffness, muscle weakness, heavier than normal menstrual periods, and/or depression.

Hysterectomy: Surgical removal of a woman's uterus. In many cases of hysterectomy, concomitant bilateral removal of the ovaries is performed. The combined removal of the uterus and ovaries is called a complete hysterectomy, resulting in surgical menopause and an abrupt lowering in estradiol values. Researchers report a lowering of estradiol after hysterectomy even when the ovaries are preserved, whereas in natural menopause the estradiol values gradually diminish. After hysterectomy, some women report adverse changes to their sexual function, especially diminished internal orgasmic intensity, while others who had pain, due to uterine pathology, report improvement in their sexual function. *See Medical Factors Science Section/Menopause*

Hystoscopic Myomectomy: Removal of fibroid tumors through the cervix using an instrument called a resectoscope. This is a surgical device with a built-in wire loop that uses high-frequency electrical energy to cut or coagulate the fibroid tissue. The resectoscope was developed to allow surgery inside an organ without the typical skin incision. Removal of fibroid tumors on or near the lining of the uterus by hystoscopic myomectomy allows the fibroids to be removed and the uterus to be spared. This may be particularly important for women who report sexual satisfaction from internal-based orgasm.

Kegel Exercises: Commonly used name for pelvic floor exercise of muscles attached from the coccyx bone at the bottom of the spinal column to the pubic bone at the front of the pelvis. These muscles act like a hammock supporting the pelvic organs, including the vagina, uterus, and bladder. The pelvic floor muscles used in Kegel exercises can be identified by the stop and start of the flow of urine. Once the muscles have been located, the woman can strengthen them by contracting and relaxing them according to her ability. Performing Kegel exercises provides many benefits, including increase in sexual enjoyment of both partners, and help in preventing prolapse of pelvic organs and urine leakage during sneezing or coughing. There are many variations on Kegel exercises. A pelvic floor physical therapist can determine which exercises are appropriate, and whether or not they are being performed properly. *See Physical Therapy Science Section*

Labia Majora: Two prominent lateral boundaries of the vulva that meet in front of the anus. Each labium has an external surface that is pigmented, covered with hair, and slightly wrinkled in the non-aroused state. The internal surface is smooth and has multiple large glands that release sebum. The labia majora serve to protect the vestibule. *See Illustrations*

Labia Minora: Two prominent lateral boundaries of the vestibule. On the top, the right and left labia minora coalesce to form the hood of the clitoral prepuce. At the bottom of the glans clitoris, the right and left labia minora form the 2 clitoral frenulae. The labia minora continue to surround the sides of the vaginal opening. The labia minora are composed of flexible, elastic skin, rich in glands that release sebum, with many sensory nerves that make the labia minora very sensitive to the touch. They commonly undergo atrophy if the blood levels of estrogen and androgen hormones are low. *See Illustrations*

Laparoscopic Examination (Laparoscopy): Direct visualization of the peritoneal cavity, ovaries, fallopian tubes, and uterus by laparoscope, a miniature telescope with a fiber optic system that brings light into the abdomen. Carbon dioxide gas is administered into the abdomen through a special needle inserted just below the umbilicus. This gas helps to separate the organs inside the abdominal cavity, making it possible for the physician to visualize and, if necessary, operate on the ovaries, fallopian tubes, and uterus or other organs such as the bladder or loops of bowel.

Libido: Sexual desire or interest for sexual activity. The opposite of hypoactive sexual desire disorder, sexual desire would therefore be the presence of, desire for, receptivity to and/or thoughts or fantasies about sexual activity. Desire is a "psychological" sexual interest in which an individual "wants" or "craves" sexual activity.

Menopause: Time of a woman's last menstrual period, when levels of estrogen and progesterone stop being produced by the ovaries. Symptoms can begin during peri-menopause, several years before menopause. Such symptoms include: changes in menstrual periods, hot flashes, night sweats, difficulty sleeping, early waking, moodiness, irritability, depression, thinning of the skin, enlarging waist line, loss of muscle, memory problems, and stiff and achy joints. Menopause lasts for one year after the last menses. Post-menopause follows menopause and lasts the rest of a woman's life. Menopause can happen any time after the age of 30, but the average age is 51. Smoking leads to earlier menopause. Surgical removal of both ovaries causes menopausal symptoms to begin immediately and is known as surgical menopause.

The genital sexual health concerns of menopause are related primarily to lowered estradiol blood levels. Diminished estradiol levels can cause the genital area to get dry and thin, leading to uncomfortable sexual intercourse and vaginal or urinary infections. *See Medical Factors Science Section/Menopause*

Metabolic Syndrome: Waist circumference equal to or greater than 35 inches; blood pressure equal to or greater than 130/85 mmHg; fasting glucose equal to or greater than 100 mg/dl; triglyceride blood tests (taken during cholesterol measurements) equal to or greater than 150 mg/dl; or HDL cholesterol (the "good" cholesterol) less than 50 mg/dl; according to the American Heart Association and the National Heart, Lung, and Blood Institute. *See Medical Therapy Science Section/Mediterranean Diet*

Minor Vestibular Glands: The tubular glandular structures occurring around the vaginal opening. Typically there are 2–10 minor vestibular glands. Minor vestibular glands release mucous into the vestibule during sexual activity. Inflammation, irritation, and infection of the minor vestibular glands are associated with vulvar vestibulitis syndrome. *See Illustrations*

Mons Pubis: Forms the upper boundary of the vulva with the labia majora on both sides. The mons pubis is a prominent cushion of hair-bearing skin and subcutaneous fat overlying the pubic bone. *See Illustrations*

Non-Coital Sexual Pain Disorder: Recurrent or persistent genital pain induced by non-coital sexual stimulation. A common example is pain experienced in the vulva or vestibule from wearing tight clothing. *See Medical Factors Science Section/Vulvodynia*

Off-label: Use of a government-approved prescription drug to treat a condition for which the drug has not yet been approved by the government regulatory agency. An example is use of FDA-approved testosterone gel indicated for treatment of male hypogonadism, in a 10% dose as treatment for sexual dysfunction and hypogonadism in women. In off-label drug use, it is important that the treating physician provide the patient with appropriate information concerning risks and benefits prior to starting drug therapy, so that the patient can make an informed decision whether or not to start or continue with the treatment.

Oophorectomy (ovariectomy): Surgical removal of the ovaries. Common indications include ovarian involvement with endometriosis, cancers, and cysts. Bilateral oophorectomy leads to surgical menopause.

Orgasm: Variable, short-lived peak sensation of extreme, intense pleasure generating an altered state of consciousness. Orgasm may be induced by physical stimulation of varied anatomic areas such as the peri-urethral glans, breast/nipple or mons, or by mental stimulation such as mental-imagery, fantasy or hypnosis. Orgasm is usually initiated by involuntary, recurring contractions of the pelvic floor muscles, especially the fibers surrounding the vagina. Orgasm is also often accompanied by rhythmic contractions of the uterus and anal region. It is associated with a significant increase in pulse and blood pressure. During orgasm, some individuals have difficulty relaxing the pelvic floor muscles after they have been repeatedly contracting. After orgasm resolves, the sexually induced genital tissue engorgement and vasocongestion passes, usually with a feeling of wellbeing and contentment. Many researchers believe that ejaculation of fluid from the female prostate accompanies orgasm.

Women may experience several kinds of orgasm: internal (deep stimulation-related), external (clitoral and vestibular-related), and blended (or a combination of the two). Internal orgasms are not associated with vaginal muscle contractions but accompanied by change in breathing activated during coitus alone and largely due to cervix contact. External orgasms are activated by either clitoral stimulation during foreplay or by clitoral stimulation during coitus and are associated with rhythmic contractions of the vagina. Blended orgasms contain elements of both external and internal orgasm.

Orgasmic Disorder: Persistent or recurrent difficulty, delay in or absence of attaining orgasm, following sufficient sexual stimulation and arousal that causes personal distress.

Ovariectomy: *See oophorectomy*

Pelvic Floor Muscles: Group of muscles spanning the underlying surface of the bony pelvis. These muscles originate at the pubis just above the genitals and extend back to the coccyx or "tailbone," forming the floor of the pelvis. Weakness of the pelvic floor muscles can lead to sexual health problems, especially prolapse of pelvic organs into the vagina. Excessive pelvic floor muscle tone may adversely affect sexual health, in particular, sexual pain. *See Physical Therapy Science Section*

Penile Implant: *See Medical Factors Science Section/Male Partner's Sexual Health*

Peri-Menopause: Time leading up to menopause. Many different symptoms of variable intensity occur during peri-menopause, including altered menstrual periods, hot flashes, and night sweats. During peri-menopause, the blood levels of estradiol and progesterone fall. In many women, the progesterone levels decrease faster than estradiol, resulting in a relatively estradiol-rich and progesterone-poor state during peri-menopause. *See Medical Factors Science Section/Menopause*

Persistent Genital Arousal Disorder (PGAD/Persistent Sexual Arousal Syndrome/PSAS): A sub-classification of female sexual arousal disorder, defined as feelings of spontaneous, persistent, and intense arousal with or without orgasm, with or without genital engorgement, in the absence of sexual desire. Persistent genital arousal disorder, formerly known as persistent sexual arousal syndrome, is an uncommon sexual health problem that can significantly interfere with a woman's overall quality of life. The spontaneous, intrusive, and unwanted genital arousal and sexual tension (e.g., tingling, throbbing, pulsating) lead some persistent genital arousal disorder victims to become humiliated, confused, isolated, frustrated, self-conscious, and shamed. There are currently no recognized safe and effective treatments that cure persistent genital arousal disorder, leading some victims to consider suicide. The current nomenclature, persistent genital arousal disorder emphasizes that women with this disorder are not sexually aroused. *See Medical Factors Science Section/Persistent Genital Arousal Disorder*

Phimosis: Condition in which the clitoral hood or prepuce cannot be retracted to expose the underlying glans clitoris. Since the area under the hood cannot be exposed, an infection may occur in this closed compartment. When medical management cannot resolve infection, dorsal slit surgery can be performed under local or regional anesthesia to remove a portion of the prepuce, thus opening the closed compartment.

Phosphodiesterase type 5 inhibitor (PDE5 Inhibitor): Oral medication, such as sildenafil (Viagra™), tadalafil (Cialis™) or vardenafil (Levitra™) that inhibits the PDE5 enzyme in genital tissues. In a woman with normal hormone values, genital tissue changes include enhanced genital tissue smooth muscle relaxation, accumulation of blood, and engorgement. In the presence of sexual stimulation, use of a PDE5 inhibitor medication would theoretically facilitate the woman's genital tissue arousal response. *See Medical Therapy Science Section/Phosphodiesterase Type 5 Inhibitor Therapy*

Progesterone: Twenty-one carbon sex steroid or hormone, produced primarily by the ovaries and adrenal glands. Progesterone is critical during the reproductive years, as it has a direct effect on the uterus and is a prerequisite for normal menstrual cycling and achieving pregnancy. The primary action of progesterone is likely on the brain's regulation of sexual activity. In the hypothalamus, progesterone appears to regulate mood and sexual behavior. Progesterone does not appear to have any appreciable effect on genital tissue structure and function, nor does it have any appreciable conversion to either androgen or estrogen. If systemic estradiol therapy is used in a menopausal woman who still has her uterus, progesterone is required as an anti-estrogen to prevent endometrial thickening, bleeding, and endometrial cancer. *See Medical Therapy Science Section/Progesterone Therapy*

Q-tip Test: Use of a cotton swab as part of the physical examination to assess the health of the vestibule in a woman with sexual health concerns. The examiner gently presses the swab at multiple locations around the labial-hymenal junction to assess for tenderness of the minor vestibular glands. Women who have significant discomfort during Q-tip testing may be considered to have vulvar vestibulitis syndrome. *See Medical Factors Science Section/Vulvodynia*

Sexual Arousal Disorder: Persistent or recurrent inability to attain or maintain sufficient sexual excitement that causes personal distress. Women with sexual arousal disorder may have sexual complaints of diminished vaginal lubrication, increased time for arousal, diminished vaginal and clitoral sensation, and difficulty with orgasm. These clinical conditions may exist, in part, due to disruptions in the normal vascular, neural, and/or endocrine regulatory mechanisms, with associated changes in genital tissue structure or cellular organization. Chronic disease states such as hypertension, atherosclerosis, diabetes, physical trauma, endocrine imbalances or medications that adversely affect genital blood flow or sensation, will contribute to genital arousal dysfunction.

Sebum: Proteinaceous secretion (usually white-yellow in color) from the skin sebaceous glands. Sebum production is usually under the control of androgens. Sebum can accumulate in a closed compartment, such as under a clitoral hood that cannot be retracted to expose the underlying glans clitoris (phimosis). Such accumulated material is called smegma.

Selective Serotonin Reuptake Inhibitor (SSRI): Increases brain levels of the neurotransmitter serotonin, a central sexual inhibitory neurotransmitter. Selective serotonin reuptake inhibitors (e.g., fluoxetine) are commonly prescribed for the safe and effective treatment of depression. SSRI users have lowered testosterone levels and reduced dopamine, a central sexual excitatory neurotransmitter. The sexual side effects of selective serotonin reuptake inhibitors are significant, including lowered sexual interest and arousal, and delayed, reduced or absent orgasm. The sexual side effects may occur in 15% to 70% of selective serotonin reuptake inhibitor users. *See Medical Factors Science Section/Anti-Depressants*

Sexual Aversion Disorder: Persistent or recurrent phobic aversion to and avoidance of sexual contact with a sexual partner that causes personal distress. Aversion is a more significant reaction in women with low sexual interest.

Sex Hormone Binding Globulin (SHBG): Protein in the circulation that binds sex steroids, especially testosterone. The physiologic action of sex hormone binding globulin is to store sex steroids in the blood. Only the "unbound" fraction of testosterone is physiologically active and enters the cells to elicit the biological response. Increases in sex hormone binding globulin, often as a result of increases in estrogen or birth control pill use, contribute to androgen insufficiency syndrome and sexual health concerns in women. *See Medical Therapy Science section/Androgen Therapy*

Sexual Pain Disorders: Include dyspareunia, non-coital sexual pain, vaginismus, and vulvodynia. *See Medical Factors Science Section/Vulvodynia*

Skene's Glands: *See Female Prostate*

Steroid Block: Administration of a mixture of steroids and anesthetic agents to help women with pain secondary to nerve damage, such as pudendal neuropathy. The mixture is injected near the tender nerve region. *See Medical Factors Science Section/Vulvodynia*

Steroid Cream, Ultra-potent: Topical treatment for itching, redness, dryness, inflammation, and discomfort of vulvar skin conditions, including lichen sclerosus, lichen planus, lichen simplex chronicus or contact dermatitis. Women who have dermatologic vulvar conditions that are treated effectively with an ultra-potent steroid cream (e.g., clobetasol) require long-term clinical follow-up. *See Medical Factors Science Section/Vulvodynia*

Testosterone: Sex steroid androgen commonly used in androgen therapy. The effects of testosterone (transdermal, topical gel or patch) on the sexual function of women have been evaluated in placebo-controlled, randomized, clinical trials. Transdermal testosterone has been reported to significantly improve sexual motivation, thoughts and fantasies of sexual activity, frequency of sexual activity, pleasure, orgasm, and satisfaction. In addition to the positive effects on sexual function, testosterone significantly improves patient wellbeing. Side effects at the dose used clinically include acne and hair growth. *See Medical Therapy Science Section/Androgen Therapy*

Total Testosterone: Records the combined portions of testosterone that are "unbound," tightly bound to the protein sex hormone binding globulin, and loosely bound to the protein albumin. Total testosterone levels are not clinically useful in women who have elevated sex hormone binding globulin levels, such as from the birth control pill, since the majority of the total testosterone will be "bound" and not physiologically available. *See Medical Therapy Science Section/Androgen Therapy*

"Unbound" Testosterone: *See Free Testosterone*

Urethral Meatus (Peri-Urethral Glans): Opening through which urine is expelled. It is located approximately 1 inch below the clitoral glans and above the vaginal opening in the midline of the vestibule. The appearance varies from a small vertical slit, to a crescent form, to a round opening. The tissue surrounding the urethral meatus is rich in sensory skin receptors, especially stretch receptors, and is an important sexual organ in women. *See Illustrations*

Vagina: Fibromuscular tube that begins at the vaginal opening below the urethral meatus. The vagina terminates where the uterine cervix projects into the inner end of the tube, forming a circular recessed space. The vaginal upper wall covers the female prostate and urethra, and is thought to be particularly sensitive during sexual activity. The vaginal lower wall covers the rectum. The vaginal tube consists of a folded, smooth lining layer called the epithelium. Underneath is a blood vessel filled layer that is the source of vaginal lubrication. Below the blood vessel layer is the smooth muscle layer that consists of an inner layer of circular-oriented muscle and an outer, thicker layer of longitudinal-oriented muscle. During penetrative sexual intercourse, the vagina envelops the erect penis. The vaginal walls can constrict and dilate due to the presence of smooth muscles and fibroelastic tissue. *See Illustrations*

Vaginal Lubrication: Consequence of increased vaginal blood flow during sexual arousal. The vaginal fluid is plasma that "leaks" out of the capillaries in the vaginal lamina propria layer and passes to the epithelial inner lining layer. The lubrication fluid accumulating on the vaginal surface is clear, slippery, and smooth, and acts to moisten the vagina. There are no glands in the vaginal tissue per se that release lubrication during sexual arousal.

Vaginismus: A painful and often prolonged contraction of the pelvic floor muscles surrounding the vagina in response to the vulva or vagina being touched.

Vaginitis: Inflammation of the vagina. Vaginitis is usually a consequence of the vaginal pH not being acidic (e.g., 4.0) but being neutral or basic (e.g., 7.5). The acidic vaginal pH acts to control the overgrowth of vaginal organisms, such as bacteria and yeast.

Vascular Insufficiency: Diminished arterial inflow. Reduced arterial blood to the vaginal and clitoral tissues can be an early warning sign of a systemic problem with the blood vessel lining layer. Low blood flow can lead to fibrosis and decreased smooth muscle of the clitoral and vaginal tissues. The symptoms of reduced blood flow are consistent with decreased genital arousal and lubrication.

Vasodilator: Causes relaxation of the walls of the blood vessels allowing increased blood flow.

Vestibular Adenitis: *See Vulvar Vestibulitis Syndrome*

Vestibular Glands: Tubular glands lining the vaginal opening that release mucous lubrication during sexual stimulation. There are approximately 2–10 minor vestibular glands. There are 2 major vestibular glands, the right and left Bartholin's glands. Pathology in the minor vestibular glands may lead to vestibular adenitis or vulvar vestibulitis syndrome. Pathology in the major vestibular glands may lead to Bartholin's cysts. *See Illustrations*

Vestibule: Area between the labia minora. The vestibule is the outer 1/5 of the vagina. The vestibule contains many sexual organs, including the glans clitoris, the prepuce or clitoral hood, the right and left frenulae, the labia minora, the urethral meatus and peri-urethral glans, the minor vestibular glands, the duct openings from the major vestibular glands, the outside of the hymenal tissues, and nerves and arteries of the skin of the vestibule. *See Illustrations*

Vestibulectomy: Surgical excision of a portion of the total vestibule, usually due to vulvar vestibulitis syndrome that has failed conservative medical and psychologic management.

Vulva: Comprised of the mons pubis, labia majora, and vestibule. *See Illustrations*

Vulvodynia: Denotes generalized and chronic pain (more than 3–6 months) of varying intensity and location in the vulvar region for which the cause is not understood. The pain from vulvodynia may be due to unknown genetic, psychologic, inflammatory, infectious, neurologic, pelvic floor disorder or hormonal factors. Elevated levels of psychologic distress, anxiety, depression, shyness, as well as low sexual self-esteem, have also been found in women with vulvodynia. Treatment of vulvodynia engages multiple specialists and various therapies, including sex therapy, physical therapy, pain management, medical therapy, hormone therapy, and, as a last resort, surgical therapy. *See Medical Factors Science Section/Vulvodynia*

Vulvar Vestibulitis Syndrome (VVS): The most common pain syndrome in premenopausal women, also known as vestibular adenitis. Women with vulvar vestibulitis syndrome typically experience a severe burning pain of varying intensity in response to contact during both sexual and non-sexual activities. The distinguishing feature of vulvar vestibulitis syndrome is that the pain occurs at a specific location: at the entrance of the vagina just above the hymenal tissue and at the beginning of the labia minora. The classic description of vulvar vestibulitis syndrome involves redness of the vulvar vestibule and pain with intercourse or tampon insertion. Positive Q-tip testing during physical examination is a hallmark. One of the most consistently reported findings associated with the onset of vulvar vestibulitis is a history of repeated yeast infections. Women with vulvar vestibulitis syndrome exhibit an increase in pelvic floor muscle tension. Use of the birth control pill has also been reported associated with vulvar vestibulitis syndrome. *See Medical Factors Science Section/Vulvodynia*

Yeast Infection, Vaginal: Typically caused by a fungus called *Candida albicans.* These yeast organisms normally live in small numbers on the skin of the vulva and vestibule, and inside the vagina. The acidic environment of the vagina helps keep yeast from growing. If the vagina becomes less acidic, yeast can grow and cause a vaginal infection. Menstruation, pregnancy, diabetes, antibiotics, hormonal contraception (e.g., birth control pills), and steroids can change the acidic balance of the vagina. Moisture and irritation of the vagina also encourage yeast to grow. Symptoms of a vaginal yeast infection include itching, burning and swelling in the vulva, vestibule, and vagina, white vaginal discharge that may resemble the texture of cottage cheese, and pain during sexual intercourse. Yeast infections are common, and most women will have one at some time in her life. Yeast infections are usually treated with medications directed against the yeast fungus (e.g., miconazole) and are available in different delivery systems, such as local treatment by intravaginal creams, ointments or suppositories, or systemic treatment by oral pills (e.g., fluconazole).

Medical Illustrations

Lori A. Messenger, C.M.I.

Biomedical Illustrator
DNA Illustration Studio
Hull, Massachusetts

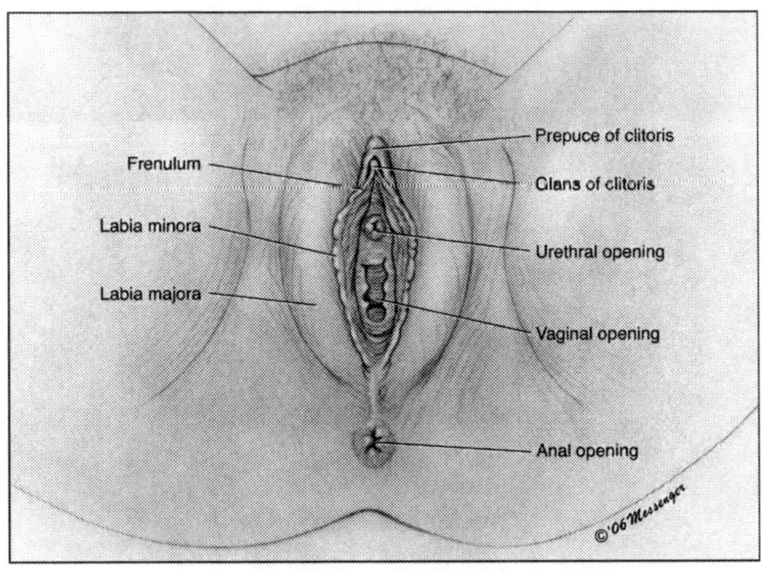
Prepuce of clitoris
Frenulum
Glans of clitoris
Labia minora
Urethral opening
Labia majora
Vaginal opening
Anal opening
©'06 Messenger

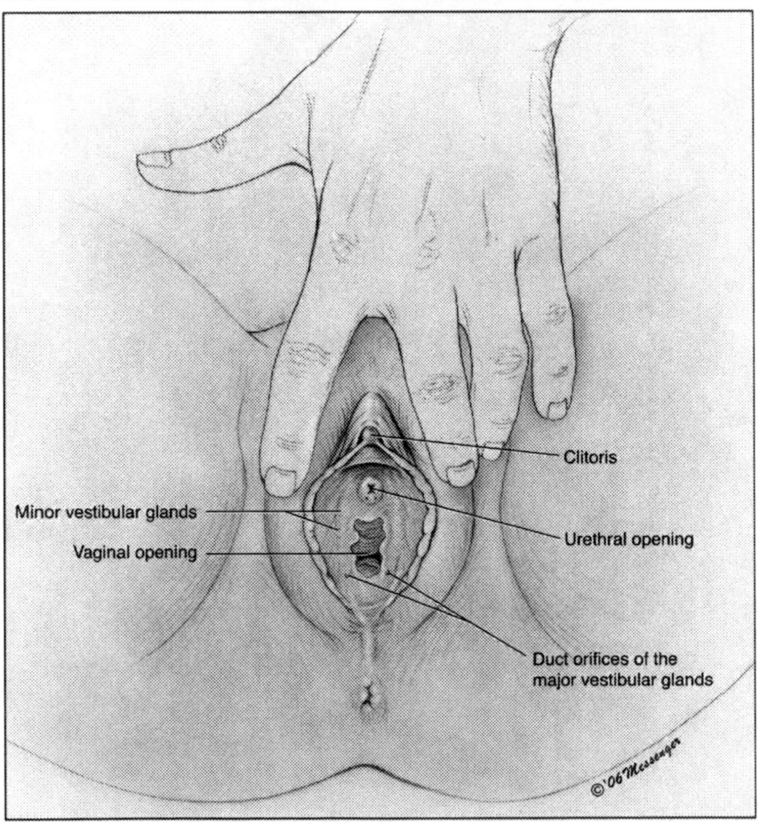
Clitoris
Minor vestibular glands
Urethral opening
Vaginal opening
Duct orifices of the
major vestibular glands
©'06 Messenger

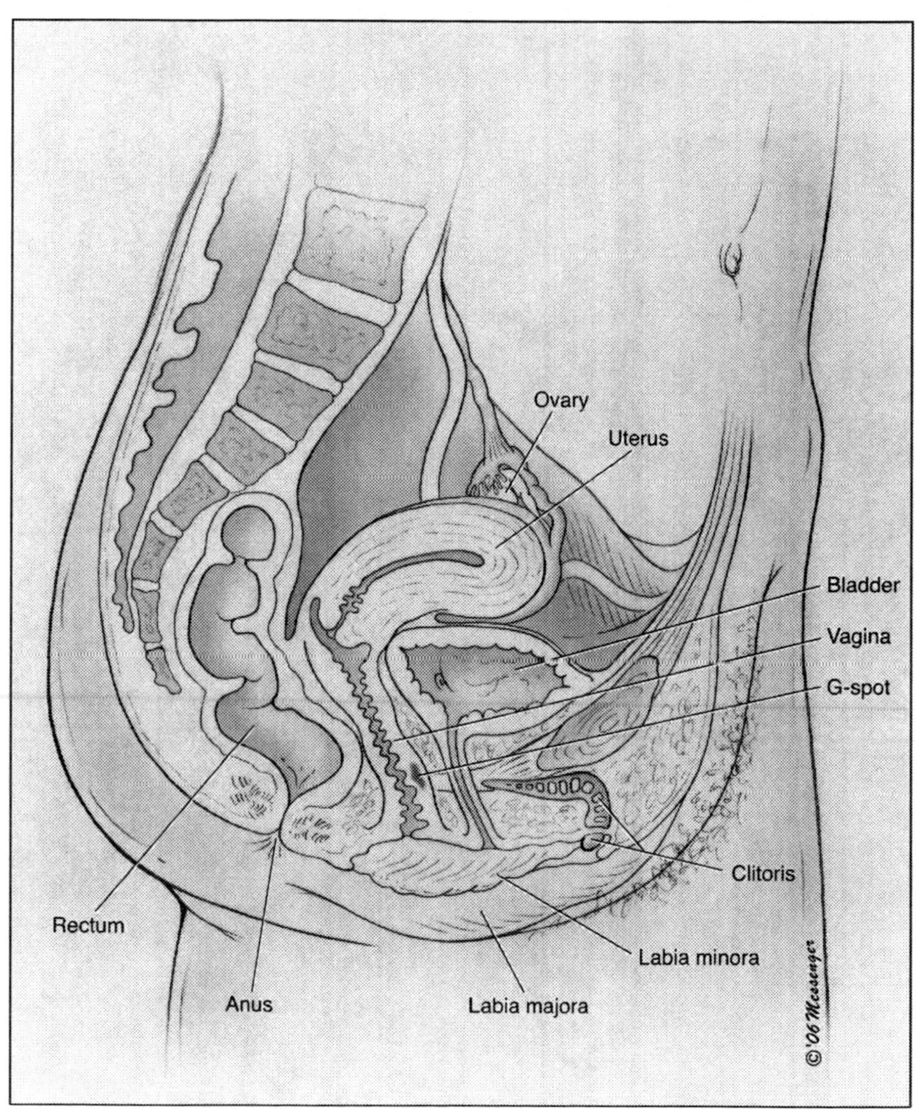

(Above) Sagittal view of a woman's internal genitalia.

(Left) Perineal view of a woman's genitalia.

Healthcare Provider Resource Page

Publications and Web Sites:

Women's Sexual Function and Dysfunction: Study, Diagnosis and Treatment
Irwin Goldstein, Cindy M. Meston, Susan R. Davis and Abdulmaged M. Traish, Editors, Taylor and Francis, London, 2006.

The Journal of Sexual Medicine
http://jsm.issm.info

Journal of Sex and Marital Therapy
http://www.tandf.co.uk/journals/titles/0092623X.asp

Archives of Sexual Behavior
http://www.ingentaconnect.com/content/klu/aseb

Irwin Goldstein, MD
http://www.irwingoldsteinmd.com

When Sex Isn't Good
http://www.whensexisntgood.com

Societies and Organizations:

International Society for the Study of Women's Sexual Health (ISSWSH)
http://www.isswsh.org

National Vulvodynia Association (NVA)
www.nva.org

International Society for Sexual Medicine (ISSM)
http://www.issm.info/

Asia Pacific Society for Sexual Medicine (APSSM)
http://www.apsir.org

European Society for Sexual Medicine (ESSM)
http://www.essm.org

Latin America Society for Sexual Medicine (SLAMS)
http://www.slamsnet.org/

Sexual Medicine Society of North America (SMSNA)
http://www.smsna.org

978-0-595-42646-1
0-595-42646-8

Printed in the United States
78514LV00003B/1-93